All about Arthritis

All about Arthritis

PAST

PRESENT

FUTURE

Derrick Brewerton

Harvard University Press

Cambridge, Massachusetts

London, England

1992

Library of Congress Cataloging-in-Publication Data

Brewerton, Derrick.
    All about arthritis: past, present, future / Derrick Brewerton.
      p. cm.
    Includes bibliographical references and index.
    ISBN 0–674–01615–7
    1. Arthritis—Popular works.   I. Title.
RC933.B73   1992
616.7'22—dc20

    92–11557
    CIP

To my father, an engineer with a flair for invention,
who taught me when a small child to understand how
scientific discoveries are made; and to Harold Geggie,
a general practitioner in the rural village of
Wakefield, Quebec, who taught me when a student to love medicine

Contents

All about Arthritis

Prologue

Physicians are not supposed to have favorites, but they do. Two of mine are Jane, a young teacher, and her husband, Philip, a design engineer. When I first met them, they had two small children and lived in a cottage with a large garden. Although Jane had had arthritis for only a few years, she was no longer able to continue her teaching, do the housework, or tend the garden. She suffered considerable pain and disability, which, like most people with arthritis, she endured with remarkable courage. Shortly after that first visit, at a time when her pain had become particularly severe, Philip came with her to the consultation. From his description it was not difficult to picture Jane sitting in the center of the parlor while their children played on the floor—choking back tears of frustration because she could not chase after them or pick them up to hug them.

That second visit was obviously important for them. They came armed with many questions about the disease that was destroying the quality of their lives and threatening the future of their family. Both had read books on the subject, but now they wished to know more, especially about the scientific aspects of arthritis. Almost inevitably, they were soon asking about the causes, about recent advances in research, and about the prospects for prevention and treatment. What I told them was clearly not enough, and soon Jane said, "Doctor, why don't you write a book—all about arthritis—one that I can understand? I would love to learn more of the things that you know and take for granted: the scientific background, the people who make the discoveries, and how soon the causes will be found."

Prompted partly by her suggestion and partly by subsequent comments from many people who do not have arthritis, I have written this book. It is about microbes, genes, molecules, and diseases; but, far more, it is about people—especially those, great and small, who have made contributions to medical research, and those who go through life with arthritis as a constant companion.

Arthritis is a human scourge. If we take a strict definition of the term and include only those people who have true inflammation of the joints resembling rheumatoid arthritis on medical examination, one adult in fifty will have definite evidence of pain, swelling, or deformity. That represents 5 million people in the United States alone. Arthritis attacks all ages—from early childhood to old age. It is common in every country, in every ethnic group, and in every level of society. In England, joint disorders result in 15 percent of all complaints to doctors and cause 40 percent of all severe physical disabilities. Worldwide, over 100 million people suffer from arthritis. The type of arthritis varies from place to place, but its frequency is approximately the same everywhere. It is a massive problem.

Attitudes toward joint diseases are complex and often ambivalent, for arthritis is encircled by ignorance and prejudice. Only those who study these common diseases and attend scientific meetings on the subject are fully aware of the exciting advances presently being made. Unfortunately, the true facts about arthritis are seldom explained to the general public; they are usually kept hidden as if in a secret society. It is no surprise, therefore, that misconceptions abound.

Despite the prevalence of arthritis in childhood (requiring a separate subspecialty of pediatric rheumatology) and the frequent occurrence of severe arthritis in adolescents and young adults, it is often believed that arthritis is a condition that affects only old people. And even though many sufferers respond dramatically to treatment, arthritis is widely considered to be incurable. It is, perhaps, more comfortable to think that arthritis is a dull, untreatable condition of the elderly about which nothing is known.

Finally, we come to the most subtle prejudice of all. Although virtually everyone would deny it, deep down we have a repressed belief that disabled people, including those with arthritis, are somehow inferior—a belief that imperceptibly spreads to include those who worry about people with arthritis or look after them. A moment's thought confirms that this concept is complete nonsense, and that people with disabilities or arthritis are just as intelligent, educated, and perceptive as anyone else; nevertheless, this prejudice leads to the view that only those suffering from arthritis would be interested in reading about it, and that they could not be expected to appreciate the scientific aspects of their disorder. Why not?

Lack of information is widespread among the vast numbers of us who have a personal interest in arthritis. Two-thirds of adults in developed countries have a relative, friend, or acquaintance afflicted with arthritis. All adults experience pain in their joints at some time, and one-third of us have enough joint symptoms to make us believe that we have arthritis. After middle age everyone has demonstrable wearing and stiffness of joints. Among these individuals with a special interest in arthritis, we encounter powerful ambivalent attitudes. Not understanding the subject—or what is known about it—people become embarrassed and frustrated. They would like to help others, or themselves, but instead they often adopt bizarre behavior patterns, even making arthritis the subject of jokes or suggesting inappropriate remedies. What they really want is to learn more about the subject.

Because scientific facts about the causes of arthritis have not been readily available, a whole world of mystique, folklore, and passionate beliefs has evolved. Arthritis and rheumatism compete with the weather and politics as topics of conversation; and many billions of dollars are spent each year on remedies that have no scientific foundation. The attachment to these beliefs and to these remedies is so strong that physicians often feel obliged to collude with the general public rather than risk confrontation on these issues. Perhaps that is a major reason why no popular, factual account concerning the causes of these diseases has been written.

As a clinical rheumatologist, I have spent most of each working day for many years listening to the problems of people with arthritis and their relatives, doing my best to provide frank answers to their queries. I know that many people with arthritis could understand the scientific facts about their disease if these facts were available in an accessible form. To my regret, I have never succeeded in replying satisfactorily to questions about the causes of arthritis—mainly because the subject is not simple and thus does not lend itself to easy answers. I owe these individuals a better response and I will try here to answer as many of their questions as I can.

When I started to write this book, I knew from the beginning that it would be impossible to be comprehensive: I decided to restrict clinical descriptions to those types of arthritis that are common, and hence will be recognized by those who suffer from them, or that illustrate a point about causation. Each year thousands of scientific publications appear on the subject of arthritis. A single textbook may contain two thousand pages and ten thousand references, weigh several pounds, and cost a small fortune. Scrupulous selection has been essential. I decided to concentrate on the *causes* of arthritis, excluding consequences, complications, and treatments. Too often in the history of medicine, doctors and scientists have devoted their energies to studying the intricate processes that follow the onset of disease in the hope that this path would lead them back to the causes. The result is usually confusion. With few exceptions, it is not until the causes are known that the disease processes, complications, and correct treatment are understood.

My next problem was how to present the necessary scientific information in as attractive a way as possible to enable readers to grasp the contents. My first decision was that structurally this book should resemble a detective story and be as little like a textbook as possible. Then, I elected to present scientific facts through the eyes of the people who made the discoveries. The history of science has much to teach us, for the problems of the past and the people who achieved success along the way point to the future and indicate what we may want to do next. To help me describe today's remarkable new phase of arthritis research, colleagues in many countries generously have told me about their findings, why they did what they did, and what they thought at the time.

When studying any landmark in the history of science, my first interest is in the depth of the ignorance that preceded it. What effects did this ignorance have? What were the views of the establishment figures at the time? Under what circumstances did new ideas emerge? Given the misunderstandings and prejudices that existed, how did certain investigators have the courage to accept the solutions offered to them by Nature and to challenge the establishment view? What were the personal backgrounds of the successful researchers, and what characteristics did they have in common? How did they take strands of knowledge from two subjects, or several subjects, and weave them together to create new ideas that had not occurred to anyone before? Having made the initial discovery, how did these outstanding people embark on the far more difficult task of deciding the crucial next steps? Most interesting, how did they perceive the significance of their observations? What did it feel like to work patiently at problems, not expecting any reward, and then to realize that what they were doing had suddenly changed the future of science?

After working on an exciting project for months or years, how did they explain their cherished findings to a scientific world that was often hostile, jealous, and critical? In centuries past, scientists who had brilliant new ideas were persecuted or put in prison. In later years the emotional reaction was less intense, but the innovative researcher who mastered problems perceived as insoluble was seldom popular with fellow scientists.

The emotional problems related to research in medical and biological sciences have always tended to be worse than in the physical sciences, because there is usually a greater element of uncertainty about the interpretation of results. Medical research seldom leads to laws that are undoubtedly and unquestionably correct. In consequence, some of the most valuable medical discoveries have been the subject of prolonged controversy. Worse still, they have often been rejected or set aside, only to be rediscovered decades later. In the words of Michel de Montaigne (1533–1592): "Whenever a new discovery is reported to the scientific world, they say first, 'It is probably not true.' Thereafter, when the truth of the proposition has been demonstrated beyond question, they say, 'Yes, it may be true, but it is not important.' Finally, when sufficient time has elapsed to fully evidence its importance, they say, 'Yes, surely it is important, but it is no longer new.'"

In a sense, arthritis research is a microcosm that represents all science. Like much medical science, it is characterized by a need to draw knowledge from many diverse subjects and from the discoveries of generations of researchers, and to apply that knowledge to strictly practical goals such as the establishment of the causes of arthritis and the development of radical new techniques of prevention and treatment.

As late as 1875, doctors did not know whether germs caused disease, and almost as many people died of infection as from all other causes. So that is where this book begins, with a description of life when infections were regarded as acts of God. In 1876 Robert Koch demonstrated the validity of the germ theory of disease. Then, in twenty golden years, specific organisms were identified for most diseases. After Louis Pasteur and Koch founded medical bacteriology and proved the germ theory of disease, thoughts soon turned to the body's natural defenses against microbes—the immune system. In 1883 Elie Metchnikoff discovered the role of cells in immune responses (cellular immunology). Shortly afterward, Emil Behring, Sibasaburo Kitasato, and Paul Ehrlich established the role of serum in immune responses (humoral immunology). During the past hundred years, many others have contributed to our understanding that hormones, nerves, and psychological processes also play critical roles in the body's defenses.

With few exceptions, the history of the study of arthritis is remarkably short. A disease as physically obvious as rheumatoid arthritis was not described until 1800 and not named until 1859. Osteoarthritis was not clearly distinguished as a separate disease until the beginning of this century. In 1894 came the first report of attempts to find microbes in joints, before which it was impossible to have meaningful thoughts about why joints became inflamed or why most arthritis occurred. In 1930, when the medical specialty of rheumatology began, research was primarily confined to clinical observation of people with arthritis and did not tackle the fundamental causes of joint disorders. It was only after World War II that research into the basic causes of arthritis began in earnest. The most helpful early development was the investigation of the disease within communities, without which little progress in understanding arthritis would have been made.

In 1971 a group of us at Westminster Hospital in London embarked on investigations that have proved to be important. To our surprise, by the time we published our results in 1973, a distinguished group in Los Angeles was publishing similar findings; for several months both groups—unknown to each other—lived in the belief that they had made a major, independent discovery. Using tissue-typing, what both had demonstrated was that a common inherited molecule renders those who are born with it a hundred times more likely to develop arthritis in later life.

At Westminster we had the exhilarating experience of visiting families in homes and hospitals throughout London. Because suitable genetic markers were available, we soon appreciated that we were investigating the multigenic heredity of several common diseases. I felt as though the key to understanding arthritis had dropped in my lap.

After reviewing all the evidence concerning the influence of heredity and other host factors in the people we examined, I suggested that all the host factors taken together (including age, sex, hormones, nerves, emotions, and nutrition) might determine the clinical details of the disease in each individual. If that were true, we need not continue to search for all-powerful microbes for each disease, because the environmental triggers could be nonspecific in their action; there could be many of them, varying even from individual to individual.

At the time of our findings, there was already a worldwide search for associations with inherited molecules. Links were rapidly established with a number of common diseases of unknown cause. Prompted by a deep sense of curiosity, many top scientists quickly became immersed in the study of arthritis. By 1975 rheumatologists were no longer working with a small number of dedicated scientists and limited resources; suddenly researchers in many disciplines wanted to join in. Largely as a result, for the past several years arthritis has been at the forefront of medical research.

Before long, it was known that there are inherited molecules for most types of arthritis, and for specific clinical features of those diseases. Worldwide population studies proved that the first inherited molecule we had studied must be an integral part of the disease in millions of people with arthritis. For many years, though, we did not know the precise function of the molecule, or how it might cause arthritis.

Fortuitously, at that time several relevant branches of science were advancing with extraordinary speed. Research on arthritis, assisted by new techniques of unbelievable complexity and sophistication, has leapt forward. The latest developments in genetics, x-ray crystallography, cell biology, and molecular biology all come into play.

Some of the characters in our story are household names; others are not. This is the case in every area of science. For example, two young assistants were the first to show that a crystal can split an x-ray beam into smaller beams, and two housewives played significant roles in discovering Lyme disease. And, of course, most of us in arthritis research are unknown except to our colleagues. Pamela Bjorkman, for instance, was a graduate student when she did her work on molecular structure. This heroic young woman spent eight years at the laboratory bench determining the detailed structure of the class of molecule that had excited us so much in the previous decade.

For a subject to be interesting to the layperson, I do not believe that all the answers must be securely in place. We have known for several decades that many factors combine to cause arthritis. The jigsaw puzzle is taking shape, the missing pieces are few, and the pace is quickening as the picture comes into view. We have not reached our final goal, but as more scientists and physicians become deeply involved in research on this subject, soon the puzzle will be complete, and new methods of prevention and treatment will transform the outlook for everyone with arthritis.

1

The Search for Germs

It is difficult to appreciate, and easy to forget, that before this century our ancestors everywhere in the world lived in constant fear of infection. Today, when we have a fever, it is a nuisance that may delay our return to work for a few days; when they had a fever, there was a distinct chance that by the next week they would be dead. When we are children or young adults, we feel safe; when they were young, they died. Without doubt, the partial conquest of infection is the greatest contribution man has made to the welfare of humankind. But the battle is not yet won. We still have sad reminders of that fact in underdeveloped countries, in the appalling mortality rates due to infection in wartime and in the tragedy that is AIDS.

We are taught in school that the plague came to Britain only twice: as the Black Death in 1348–1349, when it killed half the population of England, and as the Plague of 1665–1666, which killed one hundred thousand people in London alone. In reality, Britain was tormented by plague virtually every year for a thousand years, with sporadic deaths in towns and villages throughout the land.

The ravaged and bewildered people had little idea what caused so many deaths. In a tract by Jehan Goerout, first published in 1544, he suggested that the plague had four roots: "the will of God punishing wicked men, the heavenly constellations, the stink and corruption of the air, and the abuse of meat, drink, passions of the mind . . . and immoderate use of lechery." In their ignorance, individuals adopted many of the desperate measures that people today use to ward off diseases they do not understand. They tried amulets, bracelets, sweating followed by cold water, salad oil, evacuation, diets, treacles, and tonics to strengthen the liver.

From at least the beginning of the fourteenth century, prevention of the plague was on the agenda of every public authority. All manner of preventive measures were introduced. Most of the tactics were irrelevant, and many of them horribly cruel; but among them were the beginnings of modern public sanitation. In London there were orders to clean the streets and ditches, and to remove rubbish. People were to be punished severely if they threw refuse into ditches or into the Thames. From 1535 on, to deal with the refuse in Westminster, the "raker" blew his horn before every door on Mondays, Wednesdays, and Fridays, reminding the inhabitants to put out their rubbish. It was his duty to clean the streets and remove the litter every weekday morning before six.

In 1518 the aldermen banned the gift or sale of clothes and bedding belonging to diseased people. They were to be kept unused for three months, in a place where they could not spread infection. That same year the magistrates commanded the closing and marking of infected houses for forty days, "in sign and token of God's visitation." The constable reported the number of deaths to the mayor, closed and marked the houses of the infected, and arrested beggars and idlers. Because it was believed that the plague stemmed from God's wrath and that evil vapors arose from the corpses, the dead were buried without mourners.

It has been difficult to estimate the overall mortality from the plague, but a measure of what everyone feared can be appreciated in the pathetic story of the village of Eyam in Derbyshire. When the plague arrived from London, the villagers quarantined themselves by drawing a line around the entire village. Catastrophically, after the epidemic had run its course, of the original population of 340 only 25 had survived.

Samuel Pepys described the pathetic scene on his visit to London in October 1665: "But Lord, how empty the streets are, and melancholy, so many poor sick people in the streets, full of sores, and so many sad stories overheard as I walk, everybody talking of this man dead, and that man sick, and so many in this place, and so many in that. And they tell me that in Westminster there is never a physician, and but one apothecary left, all being dead—but that there are great hopes of a great decrease this week: God send it."

After 1666 the plague left the shores of England, never to return in force. No one knows why. Certainly there were no new preventive measures. Unfortunately, there was no way of knowing that this scourge would not come back. Fear of its return, and plans to combat it, persisted for more than two centuries, while epidemics continued on the Continent, particularly in Marseilles and Moscow.

How much improvement actually occurred during the remainder of the seventeenth century, after the plague had gone? The answer is that two-thirds of the population still died of infection by the age of forty, and in consequence the average life expectancy was thirty-seven years. Imagine the effect on family life among the emerging middle classes in London! Men married on average at age twenty-six, women at twenty-one. The mortality of their children due to infection was so dreadful (35 percent by the age of ten years) that they were repeatedly overwhelmed by grief, to such an extent that it is doubtful whether many of them dared to love their children as openly as we do today. And if the children survived, often the parents did not, so a high proportion of children were orphans before they reached adult life. As men were older at marriage, they often died leaving widows with insufficient education or experience to fend for themselves, thereby exposing them to merciless exploitation. In turn, remarriage following the death of a spouse due to infection often had serious consequences in the upbringing of the children.

The introduction of a regular census and improved recordkeeping early in the nineteenth century permitted a more accurate assessment of the effects of infection. Some improvement had taken place: life expectancy had increased from thirty-seven years to forty-one years (in 1840). Tuberculosis, described by John Bunyan as "the captain of the men of death," was responsible for 20 percent of all deaths in England. After that, in decreasing order, came dysentery, typhoid, scarlet fever, whooping cough, measles, smallpox, and diphtheria.

It is interesting to speculate why the death rate in England slowly fell over the centuries, before the cause of infection was known and before vaccination, antibiotics, and other specific measures were in regular use. Mortality before the age of forty fell from 65 percent in 1693 to 46 percent in 1838, 38 percent in 1900, 24 percent in 1920, and less than 5 percent today. At the end of the seventeenth century only 6.5 percent of the population survived to the age of eighty, compared with almost 50 percent now.

Since 1840 the overall mortality rate in England due to noninfectious causes has changed remarkably little, while the mortality caused by infection has decreased from half of the population to a small number today; hence, it is almost entirely because of the partial conquest of infection that our life expectancy has increased from forty-one years to over seventy-five years, transforming our quality of life in the process. Whether this change can be attributed to improvement in the social conditions of Dickensian London, attempted preventive measures, alterations in natural immunity, or changes in the virulence and frequency of prevalent microbes is unclear. It is not likely to have resulted from the quality of medical care.

This, then, was the immense, heartrending problem confronting medical research while it was still in its infancy. The responses of two inspiring men, Louis Pasteur and Robert Koch, generated one of the most important series of discoveries in the history of science. Before we review their achievements, though, we need to consider the scientific background against which they worked.

In 1827 a Dr. Clutterbuck reviewed the subject of infections and fevers in the English medical journal the *Lancet,* using the word "virus" in a much broader sense than we do today—to mean any poison or apparent cause of infection. He wrote: "Now I think the least objectionable idea that we can attach to a 'contagious' disease, is that it is one which is produced by a peculiar 'virus' or poison, generated in the body of someone labouring under a peculiar form of disease; and which 'virus' has the property of exciting a similar disease in others to which it is applied—whether in a solid, fluid, or gaseous state, seems quite immaterial."

No one reading Clutterbuck's review now would recognize the causes of fever or infection, although a few sentences seem brilliant when taken out of context. Nor can we have much confidence in one of the contemporary recommendations of the London Fever Hospital: "Mix an equal quantity of nitre and vitriolic acid in a tea cup, stirring it now and then . . . remove the tea cup occasionally to different parts of the room. With these precautions fever will seldom, if ever, spread."

The tragic consequences of not knowing the cause of a disease are exemplified in a serious epidemic of cholera in Calcutta in 1883–1884, at a time when the causative organism was first being identified. As was often the case in India during the last century, the supply of drinking water came from a tank that was also used for bathing and washing clothes. Seventeen deaths resulted when the clothes of a cholera victim were washed in the town drinking water.

The best way to appreciate the confused thinking of the establishment figures of the time is to read the *Lancet* volume of 1875. During that year the Pathological Society conducted a series of evening debates in London devoted to the theory that germs cause disease—the first society anywhere to do so. All the leading speakers were reported in the *Lancet* at length (if not in full), while the editor wrote a critical commentary after each meeting. Even before the discussions began, he wrote unenthusiastically: "The question remains whether we shall be any wiser for it. In point of fact, almost any hypothesis may be maintained at the present time with a sufficient show of reason, seeing that the majority of the arguments in favour of it must be in the main theoretical, the ascertained facts being so few and as yet unconnected . . . Nothing could be more unscientific, or less calculated to advance the truth, than the way in which some of the work on this subject has been done."

After the first meeting, the editor was still skeptical and expressed in writing the nationalistic prejudice of the times: "If merely rival theories are contested, the debate, however interesting, will be as barren in results as those in the French Academies." He remained unimpressed after the next meeting, commenting: "The part played by bacteria—which is the question upon which we require definite knowledge—has, it appears to us, been little elucidated in the progress of the debate . . . Should the debate terminate here . . . it will have served for little else than a demonstration of the many varieties of opinion that are afloat on the subject, and will have had but little practical value."

At the third meeting, one physician declared that "it does appear to me that the discovery of bacteria in the bodies of persons suffering from various infective diseases has not, so far, done anything to corroborate the germ theory of disease"; and another gave the mistaken view that typhus was due to overcrowding rather than contagion, and suggested that "the ravages of typhus in our crowded cities and our gaols have been enormously curtailed, not so much because of its diminished spread by contagion, but because we have learned what are the causes which engender it, and are therefore better able to prevent its occurrence."

At the final meeting, the battle waged on and on. When the debate was finally over, the editor of the *Lancet* concluded: "The balance of evi-

found on the side of those favouring the physico-chemical
n Dr. Murchison's striking argument in favour of a chemical
–that certain inorganic substances, as arsenic, show a spe-
ity for certain structures . . . —does not affect the counter
of Dr. Maclagan—that the special contagious organism of a
specific disease requires, parasite-like, a special nidus for its development. Either hypothesis is valid; but the one is not destructive of the
other."

Viewed in retrospect, the climate of the debates seems to have been
one of utter confusion—and of prejudice and intolerance of new ideas.

We can now return to Pasteur and Koch, the main founders of medical
microbiology. The elder, Louis Pasteur, was born in 1822, just twenty-
one years before Robert Koch. Pasteur grew up in humble conditions in
a small town in eastern France. He took his doctor's degree in chemistry
rather than in medicine, which explains his reluctance to investigate animals or human disease until relatively late in life (at the age of fifty-
five). When he started his first research project in 1847, he was completely conventional in his choice of subject—everyone was already
studying crystals—but what stamped him as a superb investigator was
his capacity to see what others could not see.

He was attracted immediately by an inexplicable conundrum: the
chemical structures of two types of tartaric acid were believed to be identical, even though one type rotated polarized light and the other did not.
Pasteur made several salts of tartrates, examined them under the microscope, and noticed that the facets of different salts pointed in slightly
different directions. Soon he demonstrated that this minute difference
correlated with the varying effect on polarized light. Like Archimedes,
he ran into the hall, crying, "I have just made a great discovery . . . I am
so happy that I am shaking all over."

From then on, no one was left in any doubt as to what Pasteur
thought about anything, or what he had done; he was an excellent com-
municator with a flair for the dramatic. By the age of twenty-six he had
established a national reputation as a researcher and had played a major
role in founding a new branch of science—the study of optical activity
in relation to the structure of molecules and crystals. For this work on
crystals he won the Legion of Honour and the Rumford Medal of the
Royal Society in London.

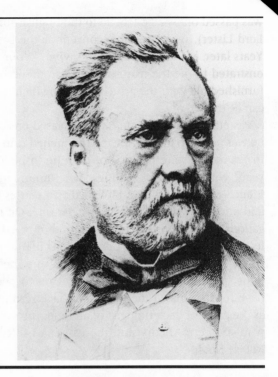

Louis Pasteur. The foremost
bacteriologist of all time,
Pasteur provided a scientific
basis for the germ theory of
disease.

At age thirty-two he was appointed Professor of Chemistry at the University of Lille. Interestingly, he was given the brief of concentrating on the industrial needs of the area, an injunction that he took very seriously, both then and later in life. It was for this reason that he was soon approached by a Monsieur Bigo, who manufactured alcohol from beet juice and was having serious difficulty with his fermentation. Many chemists at that time believed that fermentation was a chemical process, just as many doctors believed that contagion and infection were chemical processes. Looking through his microscope to investigate fermentation, Pasteur saw what others had seen—globules of yeast—but, unlike the others, he did not assume that they were innocent by-products of fermentation. Before long, he had proved conclusively that the apparently innocent globules *caused* fermentation, and that specific living, microscopic organisms orchestrated different types of fermentation.

When he published a report on this discovery in 1857, Pasteur made a totally unsubstantiated suggestion that the same principle might explain infectious diseases in humans. The significance of this comment

า by a colleague to the English surgeon Joseph Lister (later
who used this concept as the basis for antiseptic surgery.
าe wrote to Pasteur, saying, "Your brilliant researches dem-
) me the truth of the germ theory of putrefaction, and thus
าe with the principle upon which alone the antiseptic system
can be carried out."

Pasteur's first encounter with diseased creatures was in 1865, when
he was asked to investigate the threatened ruin of the silkworm industry
in France. Despite his lack of training in biology, he worked for three
years with primitive facilities in a mountainous region of southern
France and eventually established two causes of disease: malnutrition,
and infection with a microscopic parasite. On the basis of these investigations Pasteur worked out a method of breeding silkworms free of infection. During the same period of his life he published the account of
gentle heating during the production of wine and beer that led to the
term "pasteurization." Pasteur went on to perform many studies that
have revolutionized medicine and have resulted in his being described
as the greatest bacteriologist of all time. But we are concerned primarily
with the germ theory and the causes of infection, and so we turn to
Robert Koch.

Some of the most important discoveries in medicine have been made
because an investigator had a simple original idea, or made unexpected
connections between separate branches of science. Sometimes the basis
for these novel thoughts can be traced to events in childhood or early
adult life. With Robert Koch (1843–1910), the son of a mining admin-
istrator in the Harz mountains of Lower Saxony, it is probable that he
would not have proved the germ theory of disease or taken the first
photograph of bacteria had it not been for his Uncle Eduard. His uncle
was a keen naturalist who regularly took young Robert on walks to
study wildlife and passed on his own enthusiasm for photography.
Later, Koch was taught as a medical student at the University of Göttin-
gen by several revered men, among them Georg Meissner, an expert in
physiology and animal experimentation. Like most students, then and
now, Koch firmly intended to devote his life to clinical practice; but his
brief exposure to the dedication and the methods of researchers such as
Meissner was enough to alter the pattern of his career.

Upon graduation Koch—at age twenty-two—entered general practice in a small village and soon had an adoring flock of patients, whom

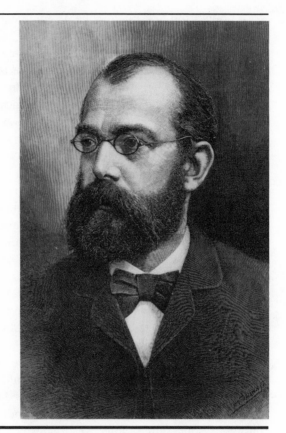

Robert Koch, Nobel Laureate. As a general practitioner—without advice, without research grants, and without money—Koch showed that anthrax bacteria cause disease and that the germ theory is correct. He later proved that tubercle bacilli cause tuberculosis.

he visited driving a horse and buggy. After various interruptions, including military service during the Franco-Prussian War, he settled with his family in Wollstein, a town of three thousand people. It was during the next eight years there, from 1872 to 1880, that Koch became world famous.

As soon as he had a reasonable income from his patients, he responded, bit by bit, to the love of research instilled in him by his teachers at medical school. As Sir Arthur Conan Doyle wrote later, "Never, surely, could a man have found himself in a position less favourable for scientific research—poor, humble, unknown, isolated from sympathy and from the scientific appliances which are the necessary tools of the investigator."

One room in the family home, already devoted to the examination of patients, was divided by a curtain to provide a minute laboratory area.

Koch bought the best microscope he could afford and set about developing new techniques for studying bacteria. There was no electricity, so he used the daylight from the window while his wife stood outside to warn him of the approach of clouds as he was taking photographs.

It was not until late 1875 that Koch began his investigations in earnest—at precisely the time that the Pathological Society was holding its meetings in London and the germ theory was being hotly debated all over Europe. Much had happened since Pasteur's publication on fermentation in 1857. In particular, a French scientist, Casimir Davaine, had studied the transmissibility of anthrax. He reported in 1863 that when a small quantity of blood was taken from a diseased animal and injected into a healthy animal, the second animal soon died of anthrax. But confusion arose because anthrax could also be transmitted by contaminated soil. At the time, "contagion" meant direct transmission from person to person; so it was reasoned that if soil was involved, anthrax could not be a contagious disease.

Koch studied anthrax partly because it was a serious disease in his community and partly because the organisms were easy to see with his microscope and easy to grow in culture. Within a month he cultured the organism responsible and transferred the disease from rabbit to rabbit. Then came the crucial connection that no one else had made: he noticed that the long, filamentous bacteria could transform themselves into small spheres. Everything he had learned from botany, and everything his Uncle Eduard had taught him, indicated that these spheres must be resting spores. Infective organisms, therefore, could lie dormant for years as spores in the soil, then reawaken to cause infection. Within six weeks Koch had established the entire life cycle of the organism that causes anthrax, and in doing so had solved the puzzle of contagion by soil. At last the germ theory of disease had a firm scientific foundation.

Like many people who have made major advances in science, Koch was overwhelmed by the enormity of his discovery. Had he made some terrible mistake? Would he make a fool of himself if he published his findings? In the end, it was only after seeking advice and gaining reassurance that he gathered the courage to publish his work. A major consequence of this publication on anthrax was that his fame spread throughout the world and Koch became firmly established in medical history.

During the next four years he lectured, improved various techniques,

and produced the first photographs of bacteria. He also took a keen interest in the development by Carl Zeiss of oil-immersion lenses for
microscopes. In order to see smaller bacteria adequately, Koch required
the difficult combination of high magnification and clear definition. Previously, there had been an air gap between the thin sheet of glass covering the bacteria and the microscope lens closest to the bacteria. The new
technique of placing oil where the air gap had been transformed Koch's
ability to see bacteria clearly at high magnification.

In 1880 Koch left his work as an isolated general practitioner and took
a senior post at the Imperial Health Office in Berlin. For the first time, he
had a research team and the necessary equipment. Two of his assistants,
Georg Gaffky and Friedrich Loeffler, were of especially high caliber and
later established worldwide reputations that have lasted to the present
day. In his new position Koch traveled and met other leaders in the
emerging field of medical bacteriology.

In August 1881 he began to study the cause of tuberculosis, the
"white plague." We know now that the causative organism is difficult to
investigate, so it is not surprising that Koch encountered problems. First,
he developed a method of staining the organism in order to see it under
the microscope. Next, he invented a new culture medium on which the
organism grew very slowly. Finally, to prove that the organism caused
infection, he took a small sample of fluid from an infected person, cultured it, injected the cultured material into a guinea pig, and confirmed
that the guinea pig had tuberculosis. He repeated the experiment many
times and proved conclusively that the tubercle bacillus is the sole cause
of this dread disease.

Once again he questioned whether he would be believed. On 24
March 1882, less than eight months after he had started to investigate
tuberculosis, he delivered a historic lecture to the Berlin Physiological
Society in front of some of the greatest scientists of the day. When he
finished, his lecture was greeted by prolonged silence. What could anyone find to criticize? Koch's work was perfect. The *New York Times* pro-
claimed his research on tuberculosis to be "one of the great scientific
discoveries of the age."

If we look back at the achievements of these two incredible men—and
consider what still remains to be done in medical research—what can
we learn? Certainly both men were intelligent, very well informed, ded-

icated, meticulous, and persistent. To my mind, the essential feature shared by Pasteur and Koch was their rare ability to stand back, review the scene in front of them, pick out the most important issue, and attack it with all the vigor of devoted problem solvers. Then, having achieved one objective, they would stand back again to select a new goal, even if it meant changing to a new subject that required new knowledge and new techniques. They were single-minded in fighting for truth; and, repeatedly, they saw what others could not see.

After the germ theory was established in 1886, bacteriology witnessed a golden period in which specific organisms for many diseases were identified at the rate of almost one a year: causative organisms for eighteen diseases had been established by the end of the century. As a consequence of this success, the discoverers (including Koch) had every reason to think that this was the inevitable pattern—one disease, one specific organism. We now know that this rule held for many diseases, but not for all.

This brief review of infection in previous centuries tells us several things about human disease. We must not be too critical if earlier doctors and scientists concentrated on diseases that killed and showed less interest in ailments that mainly diminished the quality of life. Even today we need to have sympathy for countries in which infection remains a major cause of death, and where the study and treatment of many common diseases have barely begun.

Most of all, we can now understand how a massive new group of disorders emerged. Although it had been possible to recognize diseases in which inflammation was a major feature, and then to identify from among those the diseases that were contagious, it was not until the germ theory was established that doctors began to learn about inflammatory diseases that lacked evidence of contagion and had no known cause. Until then, physicians had no way to differentiate between a swollen knee caused by an infection such as early tuberculosis, and a swollen knee caused by rheumatoid arthritis.

Inflammatory diseases that are apparently not infectious include many generalized disorders and many disorders of particular organs or tissues. Research advances in one of these disorders may be invaluable for understanding all of the others. Multiple sclerosis and arthritis are but two examples in a list that reads like a roll call of most of the diseases whose causes are not completely known, diseases that afflict a sizable portion of the human race.

In the stirring times when specific organisms were being identified in many disorders, it was to be expected that some physicians would investigate this group of diseases. Today we can look back at almost a hundred years of attempts to identify the organisms that cause these inflammatory conditions. Even though the techniques that are now used are unbelievably sensitive, and in some instances our efforts have been successful, the results in general have been deeply discouraging. If Pasteur and Koch were alive today, they would undoubtedly be looking for alternative answers to these problems—and, as we shall see, some exciting solutions are now available.

The period that established the germ theory of disease also created a scientific basis for understanding the body's defenses. As long as there was confusion about the causes of infection, it was impossible to comprehend the body's responses to those stimuli. The work of Pasteur and Koch not only founded medical microbiology, it also demonstrated the need to base strategies of treatment on a sound knowledge of two principal features of the body's defenses: inflammation and the immune system. We consider these in the next chapter.

2

The Body's Defenses

The first clear account of inflammation was that of Aurelius Cornelius Celsus, who lived in Rome at the time of Christ, during the reign of Tiberius Caesar. He was not a doctor but a private gentleman of noble family who translated the works of Hippocrates and other Greek physicians. Because he wrote with greater clarity than contemporary doctors, his works survived while others did not. In his remarkable *De re medicina,* one of the first medical books to be printed (in 1478) and widely circulated, Celsus accurately described the cardinal features of inflammation as swelling, redness, heat, and pain.

The ancient Greeks believed that the human body consisted mainly of four humors—blood, yellow bile, black bile, and phlegm—and they concluded that most diseases were caused by imbalances among these humors. Accordingly, when there was an excess of a humor, Nature had to remove it; and that was the Greek explanation of tears, sweat, saliva, a runny nose, or diarrhea. This erroneous concept of disease survived through the Middle Ages and lasted to some extent until the middle of the nineteenth century. It provided the rationale for ridiculous treatments such as bleeding, cupping, purging, vomiting, and the use of leeches.

The next big step forward was taken by Rudolf Virchow (1821–1902). In his day, he was the most influential and renowned doctor in Germany, and one of the most respected physicians in the world. Although few of his research observations were entirely original, he had strong qualities of organization, leadership, and communication. As a young man, he

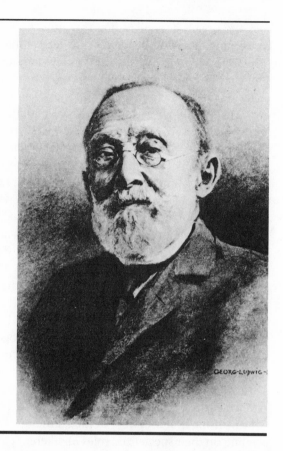

Rudolf Virchow. Virchow transformed the medical specialty of pathology, established the Berlin Pathological Institute, and popularized the role of the cell in disease.

founded a radical newspaper, wrote a report that was deeply critical of the government, and helped to organize a left-wing party. Later in life, he became a Member of Parliament and a regular adviser to government. He had the capacity to understand the social and political implications of new medical developments, and the organizational ability to put his ideas into action on a grand scale.

Virchow played a major role in the transformation of pathology, his medical specialty. (From its derivation, pathology means the study of the causes of disease and the effects of disease on the body.) Before Virchow's contributions, pathologists spent most of their time examining dead tissues and organs removed during postmortem examinations. Virchow was determined that pathology should adopt a more dynamic, more physiological approach, one that investigated the function of tissues and organs as well as their structure. As he wrote, "No information concerning the living is given by the dead alone."

In 1856 Virchow established the now-famous Berlin Pathological Institute, where he developed his theories in practical terms and trained many researchers who went on to make significant discoveries of their own. His physiological approach soon led him to champion the importance of the cell. To Virchow, cells were everything; they were the prime movers in all living phenomena, normal or abnormal, including inflammation. This belief was the core of Virchow's research. Yet he was wrong about inflammation in two profound respects: he did not believe in contagion or microbes; and he thought that cells, which proliferated so rapidly at the site of inflammation, must be derived from local tissues.

Virchow was correct in believing that cells are the units from which living organisms are built and that it is impossible to investigate inflammation without understanding their function. The human body is composed largely of cells, which are so small that fifty thousand typical blood cells can, like angels, dance on the head of a pin. Some cells float freely in the body fluids and in the blood, while others collaborate in forming tissues, in which the cells are held together by fibers and less-structured substances collectively known as "connective tissue." Strands of connective tissue may resemble a loose network, as in Figure 1, or a dense, more solid framework.

Since each human body is made up of one hundred trillion cells, it is not surprising that they vary in their structure and constituent parts, depending on their specialized roles in different parts of the body. They do, however, have certain features in common. When seen in cross section, a nucleus occupies the center and is surrounded by cytoplasm; these units in turn are encased in a cell membrane. The nucleus contains DNA (deoxyribonucleic acid), which is vital for the everyday function of the cell and for cell division. The cytoplasm contains many minute elements that are also essential for the function of the cell.

Every cell is an extremely complicated miniature factory capable of making innumerable products. Receptors on the surface recognize other parts of the body; a sophisticated system relays messages. Within most cells, approximately a billion instructions create all the enzymes and proteins that control the cell's functions.

Cells must divide for two sets of reasons: first, for development in the embryo and in subsequent growth, for constant replacement of older cells, and for special situations such as inflammation—all within one human being; and, second, to form the relatively small number of specialized cells for human reproduction, so an ovum and a sperm can fuse and create a new individual. Whatever the reason for cell division, the DNA in the nucleus provides the instructions for the construction of new cells.

As we saw with the germ theory, it is immensely difficult to recognize a new finding when current teaching indicates that your observation is wrong. How much harder it must be when you are working under the direction of a man such as Virchow, who has a favorite theory opposed to yours and is one of the most powerful doctors in the world. Consider the case of Friedrich von Recklinghausen (1833–1910), Virchow's assistant at the Pathological Institute from 1858 to 1861. During that time von Recklinghausen performed several experiments which suggested that cells might travel from a distance to the site of inflammation—with the distinct implication that Virchow was wrong in thinking that cells simply multiplied in local tissues. Again and again, von Recklinghausen was on the verge of making this important discovery, only to retreat to the conventional wisdom of the institute.

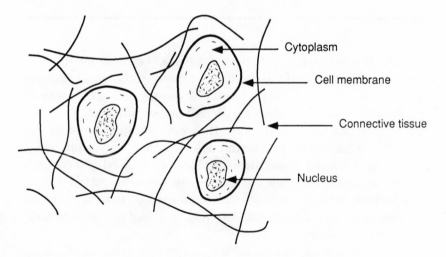

Cytoplasm

Cell membrane

Connective tissue

Nucleus

Figure 1 • In tissues, cells within tissue fluid and in a framework of connective tissue. Each cell has a nucleus, cytoplasm, and an outer cell membrane.

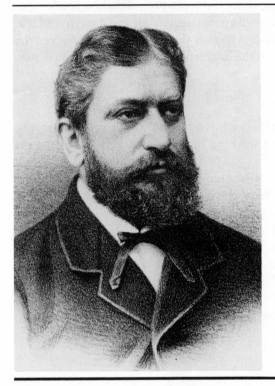

Julius Cohnheim. Working in Virchow's department, Cohnheim demonstrated that cells of the immune system travel in the bloodstream to reach a site of inflammation.

Then, in 1861, Julius Cohnheim (1839–1884) joined the institute. Prompted in part by the work of a Viennese pathologist, Salomon Stricker, who had observed red blood cells passing through the walls of capillary blood vessels, Cohnheim decided to study the small blood vessels in areas of active inflammation. He became the first to observe that white blood cells readily migrate through the walls of microscopic blood vessels into inflamed tissues. He marked live white blood cells with dye and demonstrated that these cells could come from afar and travel in the bloodstream to the point of inflammation. Even then, he reported his findings in a quiet, undemonstrative way, so as not to appear to challenge Virchow's views.

Cohnheim had solved the problem of how cells arrive at the site of inflammation but, like Virchow and von Recklinghausen before him, he could not conceive that the process might be beneficial. Before that time, very few thought of inflammation as a principal defensive mechanism. That idea had to wait another seventeen years for wide acceptance.

Just as Virchow was correct in emphasizing the importance of cells, Cohnheim was right in thinking that small blood vessels play a critical role in inflammation. To understand the implications of this notion, let us look at local circulation in tissues. You can see in Figure 2 that the blood vessels within tissues are usually reduced to very small, threadlike channels. This arrangement allows the blood vessels to release oxygen, nutrients, fluid, and cells from the bloodstream into the tissues. The linings of these small blood vessels are of paramount importance in inflammation because, as Cohnheim showed, they represent the critical barrier between the bloodstream and the tissues. Also in the tissues are minute nerve fibers, particularly surrounding the blood vessels. Then there are simple vessels, called *lymph vessels,* which drain excess fluid, cells, and proteins that can accumulate in the tissues. After passing through the lymph nodes, the lymph fluid and cells eventually return to the bloodstream.

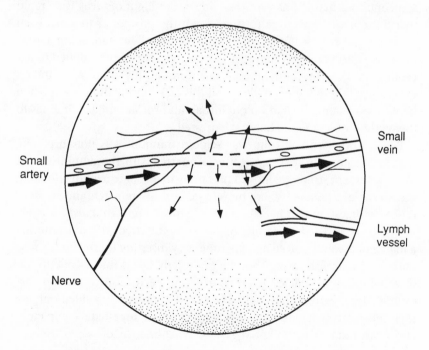

Figure 2 • Within tissues there are blood vessels, which transport oxygen, nutrients, fluid, and cells; lymph vessels, which provide drainage; and nerve fibers, which control many vital functions. The large arrows indicate the flow of blood and lymph within vessels, and the small arrows indicate fluid entering the tissues.

*　　*　　*

The next, and perhaps the crucial, step in understanding inflammation and the body's defenses was taken by Elie Metchnikoff, who was born in Russia in 1845. He studied invertebrate zoology and embryology in Russia, Germany, and Italy, and quickly became well known among zoologists. As a rising star, he was appointed Professor of Zoology in Odessa, where his special area was digestion inside the cells of invertebrate animals.

Like a number of other highly creative people in science and the arts, from an early age Metchnikoff suffered that unpleasant disease manic depression. Normally a jovial and friendly man, he intermittently plumbed the depths of despair, then ascended to the heights of elation. During his attacks of depression Metchnikoff contemplated suicide often and made serious attempts at least twice, once by taking morphia and once by injecting himself with relapsing fever. When one listens to someone in a manic phase of this illness, the flight of ideas is so rapid that there is often an urge to slow down the process or to grasp each fresh notion before it flies beyond reach. We are all hesitant about adopting new concepts, but a manic person is remarkably uninhibited in accepting the original thoughts that race through his mind. Metchnikoff experienced these flights of ideas and this lack of inhibition; even when he was less manic, he had no qualms about proclaiming his findings to the world—except when he was depressed.

Because Metchnikoff's life was seldom tranquil, it is not surprising that he resigned from Odessa after a quarrel with the administrators about a student strike. He moved his family to an apartment overlooking the Straits of Messina, where he reorganized his research and concentrated on digestion within cells of minute transparent animals.

One night in 1883 his family had gone to the circus. He was entering a manic phase and started an experiment by inserting thorns from a rose bush into a starfish larva. Then he sat quietly at his microscope to observe what happened. By his own account, each thorn was soon surrounded by moving cells. White blood cells, apparently guided only by their sense of touch, gathered around the invader, ingested it completely, and destroyed it. Metchnikoff described what happened:

> A new thought suddenly flashed across my brain. It struck me that similar cells might serve in the defence of the organism against intruders. Feeling that there was in this something of surpassing interest, I felt so

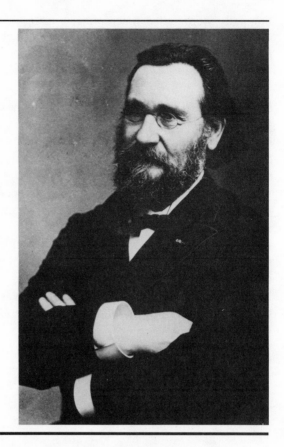

Elie Metchnikoff, Nobel Laureate. A stormy petrel of a man, Metchnikoff discovered that cells can ingest and destroy foreign substances. Against strong opposition, he established the concept of cellular immunology.

excited that I began striding up and down the room and even went to the seashore in order to collect my thoughts.

Later he reached the momentous conclusion that inflammation must be a beneficial reaction against all types of injury or invasion, and that inflammation is a primitive and ancient phenomenon that developed before animals had nerves or blood vessels.

The discovery transformed Metchnikoff's life. From then on he was devoted to the study of the body's defenses, the immune system. He identified an army of different cells that had the capacity to devour foreign substances, and he proved that they had the capacity to ingest bacteria. The whole group became known as phagocytes, from the Greek words *phagein* (to eat) and *kytos* (a cell). The big cells Metchnikoff saw originally were called macrophages, large eaters (see Figure 3). The small, lively cells he also discovered were called polymorphs, indicating that the nucleus inside the cell takes many shapes.

During the 1880s the science of microbiology, or bacteriology, came of age. No longer was it a matter of pioneers working in isolation and making discoveries that were obviously their own. Many scientists entered the field; from then on, failure to work as part of a team was often regarded as inefficient, or even incompetent.

The subject divided into three distinct branches, with separate groups studying diseases in humans, plants, and animals. Regular meetings were organized, and textbooks and journals were published. The whole world participated. In 1888 the Pasteur Institute opened in Paris, the result of worldwide public subscription. Then, in 1891, the Koch Institute opened in Berlin, funded by the German government. Later, the Rockefeller Institute for Medical Research was founded in New York City on the pattern of the Pasteur Institute and, to a lesser extent, the Koch Institute.

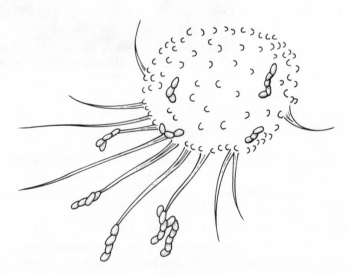

Figure 3 • Elie Metchnikoff would have been delighted with this drawing, derived from modern microscopic techniques, which shows a macrophage devouring bacteria.

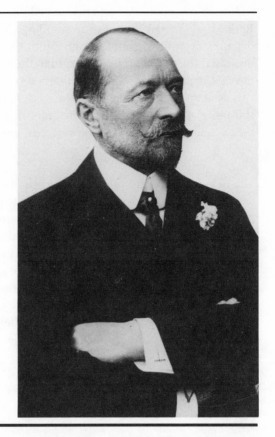

Emil Behring, Nobel Laureate. While working in the Koch Institute with Sibasaburo Kitasato, Behring demonstrated that antitoxins form in the blood in response to bacterial toxins. Together the two men established the concept of humoral immunology.

In 1884 Friedrich Loeffler, still at the Imperial Health Office in Berlin, established the cause of diphtheria; and four years later workers at the Pasteur Institute showed that the organism responsible produces a powerful toxin. By 1889 two men were working together in the Koch Institute in Berlin: Emil Behring, a former army officer, and Sibasaburo Kitasato, a Japanese who had identified the causative microbe in tetanus (and in 1894 became codiscoverer of the cause of the plague). Behring and Kitasato showed that the organism of tetanus also produces a toxin. But their crucial discovery was that when tetanus or diphtheria toxins are injected into animals, the animals produce substances that neutralize the toxins. These substances, called antitoxins, are in the blood—in the serum, not in the cells—so serum taken from an immune animal can confer immunity when injected into a susceptible animal.

Just as Metchnikoff had created cellular immunology, the group in Berlin had created humoral immunology, meaning the study of body defenses by antitoxins in the body fluids (humors). They had also demonstrated the use of antitoxic serum in the treatment of diphtheria. Antitoxins against tetanus and diphtheria proved to be the forerunners of a vast system of "antibodies" that react against "antigens"; antigens are substances that produce a specific immune response and antibodies are the proteins that respond to the antigens' provocation.

The next major contributor, Paul Ehrlich (1854–1915), had an intellect such that to call him a genius seems strangely inadequate. For him, discovery was a frequent and relatively unimportant occurrence, often arising from experimental events that were either not predicted or difficult to understand. According to Ehrlich, what mattered in research was not what you discovered, but what you thought *next* and how you arrived at the fundamental laws that governed the action you observed.

Ehrlich was born near Breslau, Germany, the son of working-class parents who had received little education themselves. His childhood and his medical education were unremarkable, apart from a passion for chemistry and for aniline dyes, about which he learned from his cousin Karl Weigert (later to become a pathologist). Perhaps as a result, Ehrlich's enduring interests throughout his career were chemistry and medicine. The study of chemicals in test tubes was the mainstay of his research.

From his profound understanding of chemistry came a stream of original ideas that transformed the whole of medicine. Although his research can be divided into three distinct periods, a single thread held together all that he did: the specificity of chemical reactions. As a student and as a young man, Ehrlich concentrated on staining cells and tissues. During this phase of his life he discovered cells that were previously unrecognized, and he made several significant contributions to the investigation of tissues, bacteria, and blood diseases. Even after he gave up this approach, he never forgot that specific dyes attached themselves to specific cells, including bacteria.

At the time Behring and Kitasato were discovering antitoxins, Ehrlich was working elbow to elbow with them at the Koch Institute; but whether he played a part in the discovery is not known. His contribution was certainly essential in the development of effective antitoxins for hu-

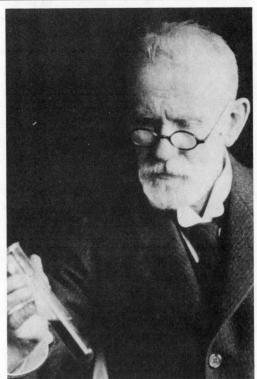

Paul Ehrlich, Nobel Laureate. Described as the greatest scientist in the history of medicine, Ehrlich contributed to the founding of immunology and to the study of cells, made many conceptual leaps, and was the father of chemotherapy.

man therapy. As a consequence of his interest in antitoxins, Ehrlich devoted thirteen years to studying aspects of immunity and body defenses. Clearly, he was fascinated by the specificity of many of the mechanisms in the immune system.

Later, from 1905 until his death in 1915, Ehrlich became absorbed in the possible application of chemicals in the treatment of disease. One of his favorite ideas had always been that if specific dyes targeted specific cells, it might be possible to identify the chemicals that were toxic to certain microbes—chemicals that acted like magic bullets. The result was the development of Salvarsan, which killed the spirochete of syphilis. Thus, he founded the chemical treatment of disease and christened it "chemotherapy."

Ehrlich was continually exploring beyond the known facts, seeking a theoretical framework that might explain what was known or that might lead to new investigations. In this he depended heavily on his remarkable visual imagination. He could see in his mind the structures of his chemicals and how they would interact; then, having produced results, he would construct visual hypotheses that provided a basis for further experiments. Understandably, he had difficulty in explaining these unconventional abstract views to others. Not being an outstanding lecturer, he preferred talking person to person, often using colored crayons to express his ideas in visual terms.

One of Ehrlich's deep concerns was how the immune system recognized the difference between foreign substances (including proteins) and substances that were normal parts of the host. He appreciated that if the ability to discriminate between self and nonself broke down, the results would be highly damaging to the host. Thus, he foretold what we now know as autoimmune diseases.

An excellent example of Ehrlich's brilliant abstract concepts is seen in the drawings he prepared for his famous lecture in 1900 to the Royal Society in London (Figure 4). He postulated that, in order to recognize foreign proteins, some cells in the blood and tissues might have specific receptors on their surface that called forth specific antibody responses for each protein; so, in effect, a receptor was an antibody. To explain how the antigen and antibody fit together, Ehrlich coined the now-familiar simile "like lock and key."

Looking back now with the advantage of current knowledge, one can only view with awe his extraordinary capacity to see the future, for it was not until many years later that the presence of receptors on the surface of cells could be confirmed by modern techniques. No wonder his views were often met with jealousy and hurtful criticism. Paul Ehrlich's lifetime undoubtedly was spent in a magnificent intellectual world all his own.

As Ehrlich and humoral immunology prospered, support for cellular immunology declined. Eventually, open warfare developed between immunologists who supported the humoral theory and those who supported the cellular theory. Few were prepared to recognize that both theories might be correct. Despite Metchnikoff's enthusiasm, and partly because of it, his extremely important proposals on the immune function of cells encountered intense opposition, first from pathologists and then from bacteriologists. After all, he was not of the establishment, he was not a doctor, and above all he was a Russian. The humoralists were

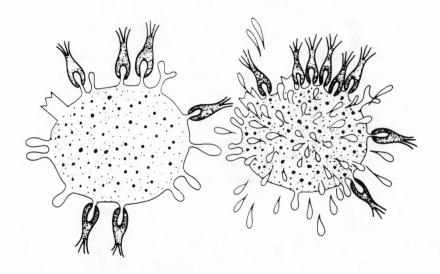

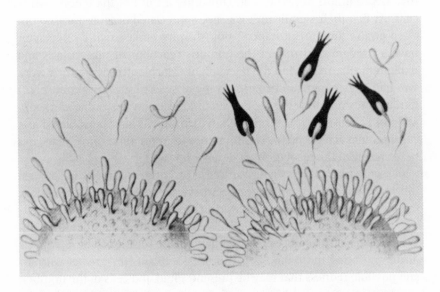

Figure 4 • These drawings by Paul Ehrlich illustrate that sometimes antibodies remain attached to the cells that form them, and sometimes they float freely and engage antigens in the body fluids.

primarily in Germany, while the cellularists were in Paris (where Metch-nikoff worked after 1888). Insults flew in unseemly fashion, and the whole debate involved more emotion and nationalism than logic. At a congress in 1891 Koch pronounced that the cellular theory was dead. From then on, every advance in knowledge about antibodies was hailed as another nail in the cellular coffin. Throughout the 1890s more and more facts were marshaled to support the humoral theory and immu-nologists imperceptibly gave up asking cellular questions. By the time Metchnikoff died in 1916, cellular immunology was held in low regard; and for at least the first four decades of the twentieth century immunol-ogists concentrated on antibodies, hoping that they would provide all the answers.

It seems to have been this emotional reaction against cellular immu-nology that led to neglect of the seminal work of James Murphy (1884–1950), director of the cancer laboratory at the Rockefeller Institute in New York. He investigated lymphocytes, small cells with round nuclei that are common in tissues and constitute a third of the blood's white cells. At first their significance was not appreciated because they do not often engulf foreign substances; but Murphy proved that lymphocytes have a fundamental role in the immune reactions of tuberculosis and malignant tumors, and in the rejection of transplanted tissues. His work was hailed by experts in America as the answer to successful transplan-tation; unfortunately, the world was interested in the humoral theory and not in cells. Murphy's research, which should have been hailed as a considerable achievement, was forgotten for more than thirty years and never received the recognition it deserved.

In summarizing the salient features of our present knowledge of local inflammation and the immune system, we see how many of the earliest theories have survived until today. In fact, Celsus' description of swell-ing, redness, heat, and pain can still be applied to acute inflammation. When a part of the body becomes inflamed, the local small blood vessels dilate and bring more blood. This process explains the greater warmth and possible redness that may be present. Fluid and cells of the immune system escape from the blood vessels into the tissues (as proposed by the Greeks, Virchow, and then Cohnheim), which accounts for the swelling and adds to the warmth.

Figures 5, 6, and 7 illustrate, at the microscopic level, the three prin-cipal mechanisms in the immune response.

1. As shown in Figure 5, polymorphs can *engulf* certain foreign sub-

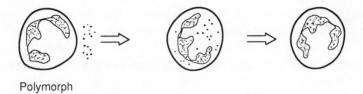

Polymorph

Figure 5 • **A polymorph engulfing and obliterating foreign substances.**

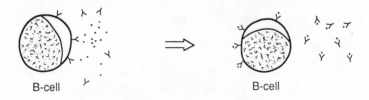

B-cell   B-cell

Figure 6 • **B-cell receptors recognizing antigens.**

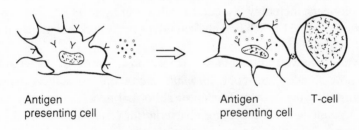

Antigen   Antigen   T-cell
presenting cell   presenting cell

Figure 7 • **A macrophage recognizing, engulfing, and processing foreign substances.**

stances and abnormal internal substances, then obliterate them (as discovered by Metchnikoff).

2. Lymphocytes, championed by Murphy, are now recognized as being of supreme importance and have been subdivided into B-cells and T-cells, which look the same under the microscope but are markedly different in function. Substances (antigens) not handled by polymorphs are recognized by *receptors* in the blood and body tissues, either on the surface of B-cells or floating freely, as predicted by Behring, Kitasato, and particularly Ehrlich. These alternatives are depicted in Figure 6. At the time Ehrlich was developing his theories, only a few antibodies had been recognized, so it was reasonable to visualize them clustering

around cells as receptors. Later it was obvious that the number of antigens, and consequently the number of antibodies, must be almost infinite. Only recently has there been an explanation of this diversity.

3. Metchnikoff was right in thinking that several kinds of cells can *digest* foreign substances, as he first observed in macrophages. The whole group has recently been classified as "antigen-presenting cells." A cell of this sort can engulf foreign substances, then process those substances and others formed internally (see Figure 7). It presents the processed material to T-cells, which in turn recruit the inflammatory response—an important process that we will consider in a later chapter.

In retrospect, we can celebrate the second half of the nineteenth century—a time when the enigma of inflammation was solved, the germ theory was proved, and the principal features of the immune system were uncovered—as the grand awakening of medical science. When the first Nobel Prize for Medicine was awarded in 1901, some of the foremost pioneers, including Pasteur, had died. But by 1908 Behring, Koch, Metchnikoff, and Ehrlich had all won the prize, as they and many others richly deserved to do.

Having reviewed inflammation in relation to germs or bacteria, we must now broaden our scope, for *many* microscopic substances that are recognized by the body as foreign or abnormal may lead to inflammation. A challenge may come from bacteria (for example, a boil), viruses (influenza), parasites (malaria), noninfectious material (silica in the lungs), a physical injury (a wound or burn), disease in a local tissue (blocked circulation), foreign tissue (a kidney transplant), a normal part of the body in an unusual place (blood in a tissue), or part of the body that has become abnormal (cancer). Any of these triggers causes the body to react and may lead to inflammation.

We have concentrated to this point on processes that are fundamental in the function of the body and in most diseases. It is time now to introduce the subject of joints.

3

Joints and Arthritis

So that the rest of the book is not like a play without a theater, let me describe the anatomy and function of human joints. Basically, a joint is a junction between two bones. As shown in Figure 8, the design of simple joints, such as the discs between bones in the spine, is almost exactly what one would expect. Between each pair of bones is an elastic cartilage with a soft, more pliable center that allows limited movement in all directions. The cartilage and the bones are encased in ligaments, which are thickened bands of white fibrous tissue that usually connect two bones. The ligaments prevent excessive movement.

When greater or more sophisticated movements are required, as they usually are, there is a space in the joint that contains a minute amount of lubricating fluid that facilitates such movement (Figure 9). This design is typical of most joints, especially those in the arms and legs.

People who have encountered bones only in a museum or when disarticulating a leg of poultry tend to perceive them as dead supporting structures—whereas in the human body they are very much alive. Bones constantly replace the substances of which they are made. After a fracture or a deformity, the bone is highly active in repairing and remodeling its own structure. Throughout life, physical stress is the main stimulus to bone replacement, which is why there is rapid loss of bone when traveling in space (there is no gravity). Loss of physical stress is also the principal reason why bones are weakened when pain and disease in arthritic joints rule out rigorous exercise.

Cartilage is designed to combine rigidity, resilience, and elasticity with

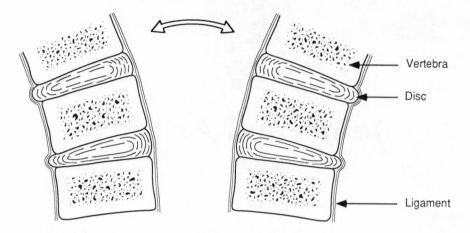

Vertebra

Disc

Ligament

Figure 8 · Despite its apparently rigid structure, the spine can bend because of the flexibility of the discs and ligaments.

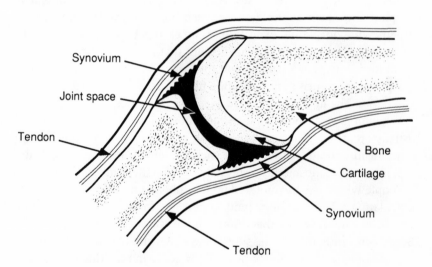

Synovium

Joint space

Tendon

Bone

Cartilage

Synovium

Tendon

Figure 9 · This imaginary section through a knuckle joint in the hand is
typical of most joints, particularly those in the arms and legs. For simplicity
the joint capsule and the ligaments are not included. The capsule is a firm
structure surrounding the synovium; the ligaments are outside the capsule,
between it and the tendons.

high tensile strength and resistance to compressive and shearing forces. Its weakness is its limited capacity to repair itself. In a disc (Figure 8), the main emphasis is on strength and elasticity. By contrast, in a joint with a space (Figure 9), the cartilage covering the ends of the bones is remarkably smooth and almost entirely free of friction. This type of cartilage is resistant to wear, despite being exposed to rapid movements and high compressive forces.

Lubrication of the cartilage surface by the fluid within the joint space has been the subject of extensive research. According to current theory, minute droplets of fluid are trapped in microscopic irregularities of the cartilage surface when it is compressed, a process called boosted lubrication.

The lubricant in a joint is a small quantity of thick, tenacious fluid. It was investigated in the sixteenth century by an extraordinary Swiss-born physician, Theophrastus Bombastus von Hohenheim, who boastfully called himself "Paracelsus," by which he meant *better than Celsus.* He was impressed by the similarity between joint fluid and egg white, so he named it "synovial fluid" (from the Greek *syn,* which means "with," and the Latin *ovum,* "an egg"). A joint with a space became a "synovial joint," the lining of such a joint became "the synovium," and inflammation of a joint became "synovitis"—as an alternative to "arthritis."

The synovium is the thin, soft lining immediately next to the joint space that surrounds it, except where there is cartilage. The synovium supplies the fluid in the joint space. From the standpoint of the causation of arthritis, the synovium is the key tissue because it is there that the disease usually begins.

Enclosing the synovium is a firm structure called the joint capsule, which provides support and keeps the joint intact. Outside the capsule are the ligaments we encountered in Figure 8. These thick bands of fibrous tissue provide the checks and balances: they direct and control joint movements, particularly in the more mobile synovial joints. As an example, Figure 10 illustrates the ligaments of a knuckle joint in the hand. These ligaments, which are on both sides of the joint, are loose when the fingers are straight, enabling a pianist to stretch an octave. But when the knuckle joints are bent, the ligaments become taut and the joints are locked, so side-to-side movements become impossible. For instance, when drinking a cup of coffee, the strain on the knuckle joints may be taken not by the muscles, but by the taut ligaments.

Figure 10 also shows the blood vessels and nerves going to the joint. Apart from important nerve fibers in the synovium, the nerves have special endings in and around the capsules and ligaments, sending to the nervous system a steady stream of information concerning movements of the joints, information that is essential to the coordination of complicated activities. The nerve endings near the capsules and the ligaments are also sensitive to painful stimuli and transmit most of the sensations of pain in a normal joint. The cartilage has few, if any, nerve fibers and is insensitive; in the substance of the bone, fibers can transmit pain if for any reason the bone loses its protective covering of cartilage.

Voluntary control of the joints is the function of muscles directed by nerves and the brain. Although muscles sometimes stretch from one bone to another, their pull is often transmitted through a tendon, which joins the end of the muscle and the bone whose movement it controls. Tendons are formed from bundles of dense connective tissue, making them much stronger and much more compact than muscle. In Figure 9 tendons that bend or extend the fingers can be seen between the joint and the skin.

To appreciate how beautifully the more sophisticated synovial joints are designed, recall the function of the ankle of a ballerina, the hip of an acrobat, the fingers of a violin virtuoso. Then, in relation to the themes of this book, imagine what it is like to spend two hours dressing in the morning because your joints are stiff and painful.

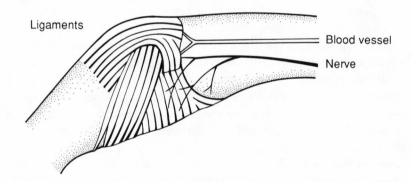

Figure 10 • Ligaments around the knuckle joint of the hand provide stability and prevent excessive movement. Blood vessels and nerves are seen entering the joint.

*　　*　　*

Having outlined some basic principles of inflammation and the anatomy of joints, we ought next to clarify some of the confusing words used in describing joint diseases. Jargon is one of the main obstacles to communication; and it is a common view that doctors not only use jargon, but often do not explain things as well as they might. In the study of joint diseases, an additional problem arises because many of the names in common use today were introduced long ago when medical understanding was limited and confused; examples of this are the terms "rheumatism," "gout," and "arthritis."

The ancient Greeks applied their mistaken beliefs concerning the imbalance of bodily humors to joints, so excess humors flowed through the body and into the joints—hence "water on the knee." It was probably Galen, a distinguished Greek physician working in Rome in the second century A.D., who coined the word "rheumatism," denoting the flowing of a bodily humor, from *reuma*, the Greek for "stream" or "flow." Thus, rheumatism with a fever became "rheumatic fever"; and a watery discharge from the eye became "rheum," a word seldom used today. Similarly, it was thought in the thirteenth century A.D. that humors flowed into the joints drop by drop. This belief gave rise to the word "gout," from *gutta*, the Latin for "drop."

Now, at the end of the twentieth century, we are captives of the past when we refer to "rheumatism." Because of misconceptions about the word, it has lost its meaning and should be abandoned. Its use is virtually confined to laypeople, who apply it to any ache, pain, or discomfort. It does immense harm to patients, who often do not know what it means, but may suffer nightmares for years because they have been frightened by the name. However strongly physicians deny the existence of rheumatism, they cannot give up words such as rheumatic fever and rheumatoid arthritis, derived from the concept. It is no small irony that rheumatologists belong to rheumatism associations and devote their careers to the study of rheumatic diseases!

"Arthritis" literally means inflammation of one or more joints, with the suffix -*itis* denoting inflammation, as in dermatitis, sinusitis, or cystitis. The Greeks, who introduced this term, correctly intended arthritis to mean inflammation of a joint. But despite their good intentions, the word "arthritis" was misused until the seventeenth century A.D., to describe virtually all painful conditions of joints, whatever their nature.

After such prolonged abuse, the word has never fully recovered. Even today, "arthritis" is commonly used to mean any abnormality of a joint or, more vaguely, to indicate minor aches and pains. Far too often physicians see patients who have been reassured by the advice, "It's only arthritis." In the future, we should resolve to be like the Greeks and restrict the meaning to conditions where inflammation is the dominant feature—and that is the definition used throughout this book.

Of all the words that are confusing and unnecessarily frightening, the worst is "osteoarthritis." "Osteo," meaning to do with bones, is not a principal feature of the condition; and the joints are not primarily inflamed but instead are worn as a result of joint failure, to which a degree of secondary inflammation may have been added. A consequence of this badly chosen name is that many people who are told they have "osteoarthritis" remember only the "arthritis" part and imagine that this dread disorder will spread to other joints and make them crippled.

As seen under the microscope, the inflammation in the different clinical types of arthritis is remarkably similar. The variations in appearance that do occur depend mainly on the severity of the inflammation, and whether the arthritis is recent or of long standing. The same processes that develop in the joints can occur in the synovial spaces that surround many tendons, and thereby lead to "tenosynovitis."

— Inflammation in a joint usually begins in the synovium. It then extends to the other structures in and around the joint. Almost immediately, the blood vessels dilate; hence, more blood flows through the joint and makes it warm and sometimes red. Fluid from the bloodstream escapes into the synovium and the tissues around the joint, and then into the joint space, all of which accounts for the swelling and sense of stiffness. At the same time, mobile cells of the immune system pass from the bloodstream into the synovium, where lymphocytes and antigen-presenting cells are of particular importance. As a consequence of the conflict between the immune system and the substances that provoked it, minute quantities of chemicals are produced and further aggravate the inflammation or cause pain.

The lymph vessels provide drainage for excess fluid, cells, and large proteins. When these substances reach the lymph nodes, their first destination, the nodes may become mildly inflamed and therefore tender and swollen.

The commonest outcome of inflammation is that it disappears and the joint or tendon returns to normal. If the inflammation persists for several weeks, various changes may ensue. The small blood vessels may be damaged irreparably, and the ligaments and capsules may be weakened and the joints loosened, either by external strains or by swelling within the joints. Scar tissue may form around the joints and cause persistent restriction of movement. Sometimes aggressive types of arthritis damage the cartilage and local bone.

Now that I have set the scene, let us consider why the synovium and the joints become inflamed, starting with the possibility that the arthritis may be caused by an infection.

4

Bacteria, Alive or Dead

The golden years of bacteriology at the end of the nineteenth century firmly established the belief that specific microbes cause specific diseases. It was soon recognized that disease susceptibility is sometimes modified by the host individual; but at that time it was thought that the person affected has little influence on what happens, apart from a general increase in the susceptibility to that type of infection. There was every reason to believe that the specific organism determines the clinical features of the disorder.

Pasteur, Koch, and their followers knew that they were only at the beginning of a search for specific microbes. They believed that, aside from bacteria, certain organisms not yet identified cause disease. And because new techniques and improved microscopes were enabling them to discover smaller and smaller organisms, they anticipated that some ailments would prove to be caused by organisms that they could not grow in culture or see with their inadequate microscopes. They appreciated that it would be a long time before they could prove that any disease characterized by inflammation was not caused by a microbe. They had to keep on searching.

In the widespread enthusiasm, it was to be expected that some physicians would investigate arthritis. The first written report is by an M. Bouchard of Paris in 1894 (although in that report he quoted more than twenty other people who had undertaken similar research). Bouchard systematically studied joints and managed to culture a wide variety of organisms. We know now that these must have been contaminants and were not related to the cause of the arthritis.

At the beginning of the twentieth century the failure to find organisms in arthritic joints led to much talk of bacterial toxins and focal sepsis. This speculation was presumably based on knowledge of the chemical poisons produced by bacteria such as those of diphtheria and tetanus. As a consequence, during the first half of the century many people with arthritis had totally unnecessary operations, with removal of teeth, tonsils, and even the large bowel; there was renewed enthusiasm for old treatments such as colonic lavage. Firm statements by senior physicians eventually ended all this unjustified surgery and treatment. The American Rheumatism Association later wrote, in a primer on rheumatic diseases, "The removal of an infected focus will not alter the course of rheumatoid arthritis, and extractions of teeth, tonsils, gall-bladders, and pelvic organs should be undertaken only when removal would be indicated if the patient did not have arthritis."

Another compelling reason why our predecessors concentrated on live bacteria is that, until the introduction of sulfonamides, penicillin, and streptomycin between 1935 and 1950, bacterial infection of bones and joints was a common, often fatal, disorder. It dominated the care of joint disease. Even now, despite the lack of evidence of live organisms in most common joint diseases, organisms do cause less common forms of arthritis and affect millions of people. So it is logical to start with those infections and review first the clinical features of those types of arthritis in which specific microbes are definitely (or probably) present.

From time to time, bacteria become established in a joint and grow as they would in an abscess, producing pus in the joint. Usually only one joint is affected, particularly a large one such as a knee, shoulder, hip, or wrist. Although the onset can be insidious and the infection difficult to diagnose, the joint condition is frequently part of a severe febrile illness and often only one manifestation of septicemia.

When, as often happens, the joint infection starts abruptly in an otherwise healthy person, the diagnosis is usually simple. The condition bears little clinical resemblance to common forms of arthritis such as rheumatoid arthritis. The joint is swollen, warm, and painful. Large joints may not be red; but small joints, as in the fingers, usually are obviously inflamed. Above all, the patient is ill.

A definitive diagnosis is made by taking a sample of blood, or by inserting a fine needle into the joint and withdrawing some of the infected synovial fluid. The organism can then be grown in culture, provided that an appropriate medium is used. More active bacteria reproduce themselves every ten minutes, resulting in a thousandfold increase in three hours. As a rule of thumb, if the bacteria are alive they can be cultured.

With acute infections of joints, diagnosis is a matter of urgency. Some bacteria have special enzymes that can cause irreparable damage to cartilage within hours; thus, treatment should begin as soon as possible.

Joint infection by live bacteria is unusually difficult to detect in five circumstances: in the newborn, in the elderly, after a therapeutic joint injection that suppresses the normal inflammatory responses, when the joint is already affected by arthritis, and when the immune system is compromised (either by disease, as in AIDS, or by treatment). In any of these situations, diagnosis may be delayed—even as long as a year—especially when the evidence of joint infection is obscured by preexisting arthritis.

In searching for causes of arthritis of obscure origin (such as rheumatoid arthritis) in which no causative organisms have been isolated, we are unlikely to find the correct answers by studying acute joint infections in which live bacteria can be cultured readily. Instead, let us turn to tuberculosis of the joints for an example of an organism that is difficult to detect. Looking back, we should not be surprised that tuberculosis became a paradigm in the search for the cause of most types of arthritis. To some extent, it remains a model today.

Because I graduated in medicine shortly before streptomycin became available and modern treatment for tuberculosis began, I have powerful memories of the devastation wrought by this disease. As a student, I drove around to villages and farmsteads in rural Quebec and learned of whole families wiped out by the disease. As an intern, I worked for two months in a large Montreal hospital devoted entirely to the surgery of lung tuberculosis. Later I was responsible for a ward of children with active disease (when I left, they presented me with a new stethoscope that remains one of my treasured possessions).

After I had completed my training in internal medicine in Montreal and in London, I decided to specialize in arthritis and to start by studying orthopedic surgery. At that time research in orthopedics was particularly promising, so I was fortunate to become the first internist to undergo a period of training in surgery at the Royal National Orthopaedic Hospital in London. There I encountered many patients with two types of tuberculosis that I had not seen before.

On my first day, the secretary gave me a long list of general orthopedic patients for whom I would be responsible. Then she added, "and here are your TB patients." It was another list of patients, almost as long as the first. I soon learned that the senior surgeons had vast experience with all types of joint infection, but despite their superb care the social consequences of bone and joint tuberculosis were appalling. Young people, my age, were parted from their homes and families to live in hospital wards in the countryside. Because the role of streptomycin was uncertain and the drug was still under trial, these people might be confined to beds made of plaster of paris for two, three, or four years, awaiting spontaneous stiffening of their joints and gradual reduction of the inflammation. Life with joint tuberculosis required immense courage.

The other group of patients comprised those presenting for the first time with symptoms suggestive of early joint tuberculosis—usually of only one joint. The onset was often insidious and unspectacular; no matter how carefully we examined the joint, it was frequently impossible to tell whether infection was present or not. Tuberculosis of a joint such as the knee could not be distinguished from rheumatoid or other arthritis of the knee.

Paradoxically, this terrible dilemma was aggravated by the advent of effective treatment. It became even more important to make a correct diagnosis and to start appropriate treatment as soon as possible. Before streptomycin, tuberculosis of the knee joint always resulted in a destroyed knee and a stiff or rigid leg. So I well remember a young woman who was one of the first to be treated with streptomycin. After the plaster of paris cast was removed from her leg and she underwent a course of intensive exercises, useful movement was restored to the knee. The surgeons had never seen such a recovery before.

Whenever the diagnosis remained in doubt, it was necessary to admit the patient to the hospital for surgical exploration of the joint and removal of local lymph nodes. By whatever means, it was essential to see the bacteria under the microscope, culture them, or grow them in guinea pigs. Culture of samples of synovial fluid removed through a fine needle was not as reliable as culture of samples of synovium taken during an operation after inspecting the inside of the joint to determine which part was diseased. Although wise at the time, this practice necessitated a great deal of invasive surgery in people who turned out to have arthritis and not tuberculosis. New knowledge soon meant that these unnecessary operations could be avoided.

Work with tuberculosis taught one fundamental lesson about joint disease: when searching for the cause of arthritis, it is not enough to study the blood and the synovial fluid; it is the synovium that holds the key. Thanks to the recent development of the fiberoptic arthroscope, it is no longer necessary to resort to surgery to examine the synovium. Using a local anesthetic and an instrument 4 mm in diameter, specialists can inspect the inside of the joint, take photographs, and remove minute specimens of tissue for investigation. The patient can walk home, scarcely aware that anything has been done. Arthroscopy now enables rheumatologists to make major advances in research, because they can study the crucial abnormalities that occur in the synovium in arthritis.

Our next concept is that, instead of live bacteria, disease may be caused by dead bacteria. For an introduction to this possibility, we go back to Robert Koch. By 1885 he had confirmed the germ theory; established the causes of anthrax, tuberculosis, and cholera; and gathered around him distinguished men who made other important discoveries. But life was never to be quite the same again. Despite the opposition of Virchow, Koch became professor and director of the new Hygiene Institute of the University of Berlin. He soon found, as have many others since, that the demands of administration and postgraduate courses were such that it was impossible for him to do any research. Eventually the stress was too severe, and he was forced to take a prolonged holiday during the summer of 1889.

When he returned, he once again started intensive research in his personal laboratory, alone and behind closed doors. The following year it became known that he had been studying the effects of an extract of dead tubercle bacilli. When he injected this extract into guinea pigs, after an interval of one or two days intense local and general responses developed. We now know that these were due to the delayed reaction of cells as a critical part of the immune response. Koch also found that if a guinea pig had never been infected with the tubercle bacillus before, the reaction was absent or mild; whereas if a guinea pig *had* been infected with tubercle bacilli, the local and general responses were severe. This was the first evidence that some cells have memories and can recognize foreign substances that they have encountered before. Besides being the forerunner of much important research devoted to the immune response by cells, the skin reaction to Koch's type of extract became a standard test in the diagnosis of human tuberculosis. Koch injected himself with the extract. After three hours he had a fever, and joint pains that persisted for several days. (My own interpretation is that this joint reaction was probably caused by impurities rather than by remnants of dead bacteria.)

Koch then took a wrong turn. Prompted by the government, he announced prematurely that his extract was a cure for tuberculosis. The consequences were disastrous. Vast numbers of patients with tuberculosis throughout the world were excited by the prospect of treatment; more than a thousand physicians visited Berlin; and congratulations poured in from many scientists, including Pasteur. But within a year clinical studies demonstrated that Koch's claims were unfounded and that the treatment was not effective. Although Koch did good work after that, his reputation had been tarnished.

Our story shifts to Los Angeles, where a professor of rheumatology at UCLA, Carl Pearson, showed that if dead bacteria (the type involved in tuberculosis) were emulsified in oil and then injected into small animals at a distance from the joints, a generalized, persistent arthritis usually developed after an interval of two weeks. This delayed reaction was probably similar in principle to the one studied by Koch, except that the joints were definitely involved. Although not appreciated at the time, it was a significant feature of Pearson's studies that some strains of small animals were susceptible to arthritis while others were not. Soon afterward it was shown that a similar arthritis follows injections using other types of dead bacteria, and water instead of oil. The common feature of almost all the extracts is that they contain debris from the cell walls of bacteria.

Twenty years after Pearson's original report, a group at the London Hospital published a revealing but little quoted article. They had used Pearson's method, but before injection they had made the dead bacteria fluorescent, so that the fragments were easy to detect under a microscope. After injecting their extract into the foot of a small animal, they found fluorescent dead bacteria in the synovium of the opposite knee. That is, the dead bacteria had been transported in the bloodstream and had readily passed through the walls of the small synovial blood vessels into the synovial tissue—just as Cohnheim had found that cells pass through the walls of blood vessels to reach a site of inflammation.

*   *   *

Thus, we have three models for arthritis caused by bacteria. In one, the bacteria are obviously alive; in another, they are alive but difficult to detect; and in the third, the bacteria are dead and fragmented. The notion that the cell walls of dead bacteria may cause common types of arthritis has become an exciting possibility. So in the rest of this chapter I consider a group of diseases known to be associated with bacterial infections, but in which live bacteria have never been identified within joints.

The first example is rheumatic fever. The worldwide history of epidemics teaches us that many organisms have arrived, caused devastating and tragic consequences, then either disappeared or become less troublesome—often without our knowing the reason for the improvement. We have discussed the departure of the plague from England. Tuberculosis, which became less frequent and less aggressive before the introduction of effective treatment, followed the same path—as did smallpox in Britain, described in 1894 by Charles Creighton: "It first left the richer classes, then it left the villages, then it left the provincial towns to centre itself in the capital. At the same time, it was leaving the age of infancy and childhood."

Rheumatic fever has a similar history. Primarily characterized by fever, arthritis, and inflammation of the heart, it is also associated with rashes and sometimes a disorder of the brain (chorea, which results in spontaneous movements, lack of coordination, and weakness). The average age of onset of rheumatic fever is eight years. In most developed countries where it was an immense problem in the past, it has now become rare; but, tragically, in deprived populations between 15 million and 20 million new cases are reported each year. Even the United States has shown a recent increase in rheumatic fever epidemics.

The association of fever with an acute form of arthritis was well known to the ancient Greeks and their successors through the centuries. Thomas Sydenham (1624–1689), the greatest English physician of his century, described the malady as "chiefly attacking the young and vigorous—those in the flower of their age . . . The patient is attacked by severe pains in the joints—this pain changes its place from time to time, takes the joints in turn, and affects the one that it attacks last with redness and swelling."

The connection with heart disease was not appreciated until the nineteenth century because it was seldom evident that the heart was involved until months or years after the illness, and because physicians did not realize the value of listening to the heart. Only in 1816 did René-Théophile-Hyacinthe Laënnec (1781–1826) invent the stethoscope, at first a simple wooden cylinder 30 cm in length. Ten years later he reported the use of his stethoscope in the diagnosis of mitral stenosis, a thickening and narrowing of the mitral valve of the heart, which was not then known to be a consequence of rheumatic fever.

Jean Bouillaud (1796–1881) was not the first to describe the association between rheumatic fever and heart pathology, but he was certainly the first to appreciate its significance. In 1837 he wrote:

> In listening to the sounds of the heart in some individuals still labouring under, or convalescing from, acute articular rheumatism, I was not a little surprised to hear a strong file, saw, or bellows sound, such as I had often met with in chronic or organic induration of the valves . . . I soon discovered that an acute affection of the heart, in cases of acute articular rheumatism associated with violent fever, was not a simple accident, a rare or as it were fortuitous complication, but in truth the most usual accompaniment of this disease.

In 1850 came the recognition that rheumatic fever is sometimes associated with chorea, a condition first described by Thomas Sydenham two centuries before, although he did not link the two diseases. Three decades later it was first reported that rheumatic fever usually followed two or three weeks after tonsillitis. As late as 1923, however, a distinguished English physician working extensively with rheumatic fever asserted, "Rheumatism is not a contagious disease."

Evidence of the influence of overcrowding and infection by airborne droplets from the mouth or nose gradually accumulated. At a British navy training establishment in 1912, boys fifteen years of age were admitted for periods of nine months' training. They slept in old wooden battleships, in hammocks spaced 16 inches apart. In such crowded conditions the incidence of rheumatic fever each year was 44 per 1,000 boys—even higher among newcomers. This appalling situation was mercifully rectified by transferring the boys to barracks on shore.

No disease had a more clear-cut social incidence. Rheumatic fever was a disease of poverty and of towns. It was thirty times as common among poorer children in industrial towns as among the children of the wealthy. The more poverty, malnutrition, overcrowding, and poor housing there was, the higher the incidence of the disease. But it is difficult to estimate the incidence of rheumatic fever in developed countries during the early part of this century. Some measure can be gained from the building around London of several hundred beds for children recovering from the disease. In the age group between ten and fifteen years, approximately 14 percent of the deaths in England in 1927–1928 were due to rheumatic fever, compared with 21 percent due to tuberculosis.

During the second half of the nineteenth century, about 85 people out of every million died of the consequences of rheumatic fever in England—and rather more in the United States. The equivalent figure in England in 1900 was 67, which fell progressively to 23 by 1939. In 1930 Allison Glover, a medical officer at the Ministry of Health, wrote:

> Every slum destroyed, every overcrowded tenement cleared, every unhygienic school building improved, every playing field provided, is a step forward. Education of parents and children as to nurture, diet, and fresh air are of great importance, and every improvement in food, wages, hours of work, and sobriety helps to raise the resistance of the child of the industrialized town against the infection of acute rheumatism.

Then, with the social upheaval of World War II, including the evacuation of children in the slums to the countryside, the figure fell to 12 per million by 1942. All of this was before the advent of penicillin.

Because of the delay between the infection and the symptoms of joint or heart disease, the nature of the causative organism was slow to emerge. Epidemiologists could point to parallel frequencies of scarlet fever, tonsillitis, and rheumatic fever, but not until 1931 were streptococci proved to be responsible. Then, during World War II, studies of American servicemen finally established the link between rheumatic fever and group A beta-hemolytic streptococcal infection.

As usual, the problem was not that simple. Years before, wealthy British children living in private schools seemed to be protected from rheumatic fever, despite regular epidemics of tonsillitis. Conversely, healthy American servicemen in World War II readily developed rheumatic fever when living in crowded conditions.

Although many strains of streptococci exist, there is no generally accepted proof that any strain is more likely than any other strain to cause arthritis. Streptococcal infections of the throat, however, often lead to arthritis, while infections of the skin are associated with kidney disease.

Also, there is no doubt that people who have once had rheumatic fever are susceptible to recurrences following further streptococcal infections.

Penicillin has brought new strategies. Recurrences of rheumatic fever can be prevented by prophylactic penicillin; to a lesser degree, initial attacks can be aborted. In addition, epidemics of streptococcal sore throat can be overcome by mass prophylactic treatment with penicillin.

Rheumatic fever, then, is a common arthritic disease with a known cause. But organisms have not been found in any of the joint, heart, or other tissues involved in the disease. So far we can only speculate on the mechanisms by which streptococci lead to this complaint. It is still not clear why—apart from less overcrowding, diminished virulence of the organism, and modern treatment—rheumatic fever has become a rarity in more advanced countries. Nevertheless, the developed world has a clear obligation to bring comparable improvement to the millions in less privileged countries who still suffer this dreadful ailment.

A different, less well known disease, erythema nodosum (meaning a red rash), was first described in 1798 by a London physician, Robert Willan (1757–1812), the father of English dermatology. At first thought to be a specific condition, erythema nodosum was soon recognized as a reaction to a wide variety of causes. The onset includes a mild fever, followed by purplish-red areas on the front of the legs (or, less commonly, on the thighs and forearms). These areas in the skin are raised, round, hot, painful, and tender—and very characteristic. Erythema nodosum is five times as common in women as in men; and it usually occurs between the ages of twenty and forty-five years. Symptoms subside within a few weeks.

Half of the patients with this condition have painful joints, usually consisting of obvious arthritis with swelling, particularly of the knees, ankles, and wrists. The commonest outcome is for the arthritis to disappear after a few weeks, but occasionally it persists or recurs. What is scientifically important about this illness is that it may be caused by infections with different bacteria that do not resemble one another, by a variety of fungi, and by unrelated drugs. It may also be associated with different disorders of unknown cause (particularly the disease known as sarcoidosis). The final common pathway, then, arises from many completely different causes. The mechanisms in this type of arthritis have not been established; surprisingly, they have attracted remarkably little interest in recent years.

Erythema nodosum is, therefore, another model in causation. From now on, in addition to live or dead bacteria, we must consider the possibility of multiple dissimilar causes leading to a single type of arthritis—the exact opposite of Koch's concept of a specific organism corresponding to a specific disease.

In times past, and certainly in times present, sex has been blamed for many diseases. Sickness in general has always had spiritual, religious, and moral implications, and it was only to be expected that adulterers would suffer not only sexually acquired diseases, but other punishments as well. So if you look hard enough in the medical literature, you will find the odd sentence which implies that sex causes arthritis. In my opinion, the first satisfactory account of sexually acquired arthritis was given by Benjamin Brodie (1783–1862), a talented young London surgeon, then working as Assistant Surgeon to St. George's Hospital at Hyde Park Corner and already a Fellow of the Royal Society.

In Brodie's book, *Pathological and Surgical Observations on Diseases of the Joints* (published in 1818), he reported on five patients with a similar type of disease. Describing the first man, Brodie wrote:

> There is a purulent discharge from the urethra . . . The affection arose from inflammation of the synovial membranes belonging to the joints . . . The left knee became painful, and on the following day the synovial membrane of this joint was found exceedingly distended with synovia. He was now completely crippled, compelled to keep his bed, and scarcely able to vary his position in the smallest degree without assistance.

Brodie added several similar cases in subsequent editions of the book. Overall, he gave definitive accounts of a disease that followed sexually acquired infection of the urethra and that comprised arthritis (particularly of the knees, ankles, and feet) and sometimes inflammation of the eyes.

This set of symptoms was not new. Caelius Aurelianus in the fifth century had described a comparable type of arthritis—following dysentery. At least fifteen similar reports were written before several authors in

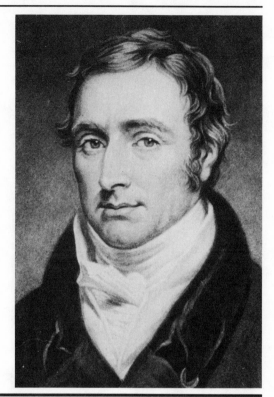

Sir Benjamin Brodie. Brodie provided the first detailed account of sexually acquired arthritis and became the leader of the surgical profession in England. He was Surgeon to King George IV and King William IV, then to Queen Victoria—who in 1834 made him a baronet. Apart from being President of the Royal Society of Medicine, he was the only man ever to become President of the Royal College of Surgeons, President of the General Medical Council, and President of the Royal Society.

1916 described patients seen in the trenches during World War I. In 1917 and 1918 two series of 59 cases and 140 cases were recorded.

In 1916 Hans Reiter wrote a case report that has had remarkable consequences. Reiter, who was born in Leipzig in 1881, received his undergraduate education in Tübingen, Breslau, and Leipzig, then studied bacteriology at the Pasteur Institute and under Sir Almroth Wright at St. Mary's Hospital in London. Later, as an assistant doctor in the German army stationed at Chauny, France, he had the considerable distinction of identifying, for the first time, the causative organism of "rat-bite fever" (Weil's disease). On the Balkan front he treated an officer with diarrhea, conjunctivitis, urethritis, and arthritis, which he incorrectly attributed to an organism similar to that of rat-bite fever. Because of a brief article about this officer, the name "Reiter's disease" was given to all patients with this type of arthritis, whether following sexually acquired

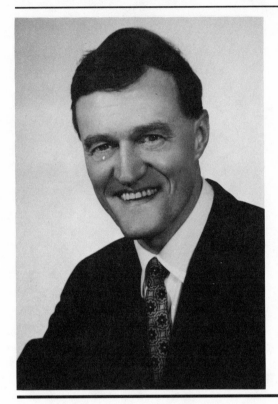

Ilmari Paronen. A Finnish physician, Paronen in World War II studied an epidemic of arthritis following dysentery, wrote a classic monograph, and provided a clinical basis for understanding post-dysenteric arthritis.

infection or dysentery. As a consequence, Reiter is by far the most commonly quoted eponymous name in rheumatology.

The one case described by Reiter can be compared with the 344 cases thoroughly assessed by Ilmari Paronen while working in wartime Finland during 1943–1945. The majority of Paronen's patients became ill as the result of a widespread epidemic of more than 150,000 cases of dysentery on the Karelian Isthmus in the summer of 1944. Paronen examined all 344 patients with arthritis at either the Thirty-first Field Hospital on Karelia or at the Fifty-sixth War Hospital in Nokia and wrote a detailed report that became a classic. Two decades later he participated in a follow-up study of one hundred of those patients. Twenty were completely free of symptoms, and about a third had minor symptoms that were difficult to assess or to attribute to the original disease. Forty-two had permanent disability that clearly resulted from the initial epidemic:

inflammation of the spine was present in thirty-two, arthritis of the limbs in eighteen, and inflammation of the eyes in seven.

We now know that different types of bacteria can cause the dysentery that precedes this type of arthritis; moreover, some strains of these organisms appear to be more likely than others to result in arthritis.

The arthritis and other clinical features of this disease are similar whether they follow sexually acquired infection or dysentery. The exception—for reasons we do not yet understand—is that sexually acquired arthritis occurs primarily in young men, while post-dysenteric arthritis occurs with equal frequency in both sexes. Only 1 to 3 percent of people with the initial infection develop arthritis, so there has to be a reason why some are so susceptible to arthritis.

Joint symptoms begin two to four weeks after the infection. In most people only a few joints are affected: knees, ankles, feet, and wrists. Frequently, the symptoms subside spontaneously in about three months. Conditions of the skin, eyes, mouth, and other parts of the body occur in some patients. As we have learned from Paronen, about half of those seen in a long-term follow-up have persistent symptoms whose commonest features result from inflammation and stiffness of the spine.

For many decades attempts to identify organisms in the synovium and synovial fluid have failed. In recent years several workers, including Andrew Keat, my colleague at Westminster Hospital, found traces of relevant bacteria within the joints of patients with sexually acquired arthritis. The work was painstaking, and only fragments of dead bacteria were identified.

In 1990, a group in Finland published an important paper on the study of nine patients with reactive arthritis after salmonella infection. Despite their inability to grow live bacteria from the joints, the investigators demonstrated, in synovial cells of all the patients, a toxin (lipopolysaccharide) derived from cell walls of salmonella bacteria.

Before then, in 1969, a different group in Finland had suggested that the term "reactive" be applied to forms of arthritis (rheumatic fever, sexually acquired arthritis, and post-dysenteric arthritis) in which the disease is initiated by an infection but no evidence of live organisms can be found in the joints. This makes "reactive arthritis" more a concept than a diagnosis, and subject to alteration with new evidence. Nevertheless, if everyone accepts its shortcomings (as they do), reactive arthritis is a more appropriate name for sexually acquired and post-dysenteric arthritis than Reiter's disease. Few clinicians would wish to apply the same name to rheumatic fever or to erythema nodosum, however, because of the differences in their clinical characteristics.

So, to live bacteria and dead bacteria causing arthritis, we can add four new principles. First, an organism, such as the streptococcus, may cause arthritis and not be found in joints. Second, many people may have the same readily identifiable causative infection, but only a small proportion of them develop arthritis. Third, as seen in erythema nodosum and re-active arthritis, Koch's idea of a specific organism for each type of disease is too exclusive. Fourth, reactive arthritis, in which the causative organism probably does not enter the joints alive, provides an attractive model which may explain other, more common forms of arthritis.

5

Tales of Ticks in America

One of Robert Koch's firm beliefs was that causes of infection other than bacteria would be identified in due course. So when the opportunity arose to prove that theory, he was fortunate in having an ardent follower in Washington—Theobald Smith of the Bureau of Animal Industry in the U.S. Department of Agriculture. The mysterious problem was Texas cattle fever.

In the spring of 1796 a herd of apparently healthy cattle was driven from South Carolina into Pennsylvania. That summer the local cattle were decimated, particularly in Lancaster County. Seventy years later, early in June 1868, a consignment of Texas cattle was shipped up the Mississippi River to Cairo, Illinois, and from there by rail to other parts of Illinois and to Indiana. A few weeks later massive losses of cattle in those two states caused widespread concern throughout the country. In New York the cattle commissioners and the board of health did everything possible to block the import of diseased cattle from the West. Because of their activities, formal inquiries were begun.

The most puzzling features of these epidemics were that the cattle which carried the disease were healthy and that the presumed infection did not spread directly from animal to animal. The carriers could be traced to most southern states and a few northern ones. Northern cattle became ill only after passing over ground previously grazed by cattle carrying the disease. Two other inexplicable, apparently unconnected, observations were that if southern cattle stayed in one place for a long time, or were driven for a considerable distance, they lost their capacity to pass on infection. Also, when disease-free cattle went through infected land, thirty days would elapse before they began to die. Just the sort of problem that Sherlock Holmes would have relished a few years later!

More strange yet, some cattle owners believed that Texas cattle fever was caused by ticks. This scenario was deemed impossible because, at that time, it was not appreciated that insects could carry infection. One expert had written in 1868, "The tick theory has acquired quite a renown during the past summer, but a little thought should have satisfied anyone of the absurdity of the idea."

When in 1889 the Bureau of Animal Industry undertook its investigations, Theobald Smith (a pathologist) concentrated on laboratory studies, while F. L. Kilborne (a veterinary surgeon) organized the fieldwork. Having shown that severe destruction of red cells in the blood was a major feature of the disease, Smith soon identified small parasites in these blood cells. They were similar to the parasites found (in 1881) in the red blood cells of malaria patients, but different in detail (now known to be the protozoan *Babesia bigemina*). Smith found no bacteria despite an extensive search for all the types of bacteria recognized at that time.

He then encountered two obstacles that made it impossible to follow the techniques developed by Koch. First, the parasites could not be grown in culture, and second, the parasites could not be transmitted to other animals. He tried in vain to inoculate sheep, guinea pigs, pigeons, and rabbits. Only cattle were susceptible to the disease.

An experimental farm, within a half-mile of Washington's city limits, was turned over to Smith and Kilborne for extensive epidemiological studies. Over four summers all the fields and wooded areas were used, and in each enclosure were placed a few cattle from various states. The researchers tested every possible explanation of how Texas cattle fever was caused. Disease-free cattle were put with southern cattle infested with ticks, with southern cattle from which the ticks were removed by hand each day, with ticks distributed on the ground, and so on.

By 1892 the research had established that Texas cattle fever was transmitted by cattle ticks, and in no other way. Cattle became infected only if the ground was infested with young ticks. Fortunately for the experiment, it was a local phenomenon, so cattle in neighboring enclosures remained healthy. The delayed onset of disease depended on the life cycle of the ticks. When infected cattle entered a new field early in summer, ripe ticks dropped off and laid their eggs after one week. Three weeks later young ticks hatched and immediately crawled onto the cattle, which suffered from fever after another ten days. To explain the seasonal incidence, Smith and Kilborne showed that low temperatures retarded the development of tick embryos, so the eggs could keep throughout the winter and hatch when the weather warmed up in the spring.

This was practical research at its very best. Soon afterward the work on Texas cattle fever provided a model for establishing the role of the tsetse fly in trypanosomiasis. It also led to the discovery, in Africa and in Italy, that mosquitoes transmit malaria. In 1895 Smith became Professor of Comparative Pathology at Harvard Medical School. Today he is recognized to have been the premier American microbiologist of his time.

Another tale involves Native Americans. For a long time the Flat Head and Nez Perce Indians in the Rocky Mountains believed that evil spirits came down among them each spring. From April to June some of their fittest young people died after a short illness—and there was no other apparent reason. The local inhabitants and the local doctors gradually defined this visitation more accurately. The disease occurred in Idaho, Montana, and Wyoming, particularly along the Snake River. It was common among men building railroads, bridges, and canals—carpenters, bridge builders, civil engineers, and so on—who often slept, unprotected, on the ground near where they worked.

This disease did not cause arthritis. Instead, it was severe, with fever, a widespread rash, and death after about one week in half of those affected. From observation, the locals came to associate the illness with ticks, but they had no real proof. Three names were used at that time: spotted fever, tick fever, and Rocky Mountain fever, the last being the one that has survived.

This formidable problem attracted the enthusiastic interest of one of the tragic heroes of medicine. Howard Taylor Ricketts, a brilliant and adventurous young pathologist, arrived in the Bitter Root Valley during the spring of 1906. By then clinical bacteriology was a well-established specialty, and the methods that Koch had fought so hard to establish were used everywhere.

Although Ricketts spent four summers in the valley, it took only a few weeks to make his principal observations. Unlike Theobald Smith in his investigation of cattle fever, Ricketts was at a disadvantage in that no organism could be seen under the microscope; but he gained an immediate advantage when he discovered that guinea pigs are susceptible to the disease and die of it after one week. Although he could not see or culture any organisms, he quickly established an inexpensive animal model, which proved without doubt that an infectious organism was responsible. He then exposed guinea pigs to ticks and proved that the ticks transmitted the disease. Next, he used the method whereby viruses were separated and identified by passing infected material through a fine filter and examining the resultant fluid. He demonstrated that the suspected organism was too big to pass through a standard fine filter and therefore was not a virus. The organism was too small to be seen but too large to pass through a filter.

That winter, at Ricketts' request, the local people scoured the area to determine where the ticks hibernated. They were not found under rocks or under vegetation as had been anticipated. Instead, large numbers of ticks were handpicked from horses and other animals, indicating that tick control was one method of prevention.

In 1908 Ricketts won the gold medal of the American Medical Association for his research. The following year he asked the state of Montana for $6,000 to develop a vaccine, but the legislature was unable to make up its mind. Frustrated and impatient to get on with his research, with tragic consequences he accepted an invitation to go to Mexico to study an illness called tabardillo, which he showed to be typhus.

Despite unsatisfactory facilities, Ricketts and his colleagues made rapid progress. By April of 1910 he and Russell Wilder announced that they had found an organism that appeared to be the cause of typhus. In the midst of this hectic activity, Ricketts was appointed to the Chair of Pathology at the University of Pennsylvania. But it was not to be. While finishing his work in Mexico City, he was bitten by an infected tick and died a week later, at the age of thirty-nine.

The short, brilliant life of Howard Ricketts had many important consequences. The organism found by Ricketts and Wilder was isolated in 1916; in 1922 it was confirmed as the cause of typhus. Soon afterward, it was established that the causes of Rocky Mountain fever and typhus are two similar but distinct bacteria with unusual characteristics. They are now classified as part of a large family of bacteria, which is called Rickettsia. No man ever did more to justify such an honor.

Rocky Mountain fever has turned out to be a misnomer. A recent count showed that 65 percent of the patients with the disease were in an area from Oklahoma to Maryland, while only 2 percent were in the mountains. Thanks to preventive measures and antibiotics, the disease can now be avoided and the mortality rate has been reduced from 50 percent to 5 percent, a figure which could be reduced still further with early diagnosis. On the dark side, during World War I, 30 million people in Eastern Europe died of typhus, and during World War II, untold numbers in concentration camps died of typhus, all due to rickettsia infection.

Let us shift to the East Coast and consider the Murray family in the village of Lyme, Connecticut. It seems that during the 1960s the Murrays complained of several mysterious symptoms, including rashes, sore throats, fevers, and painful joints. They consulted more than thirty doctors in various specialties, but no one could suggest an acceptable diagnosis. The mother, Polly, was incorrectly diagnosed as having rheumatic fever.

Because of the family exposure to ticks on Cape Cod and in Lyme, Polly wondered if their symptoms might be a delayed reaction to tick bites. She asked an internist about this possibility, but he said what any of us at the time would have said: the family's symptoms did not resemble Rocky Mountain spotted fever.

Polly continued to see specialists and continued to read the medical literature. Then, in 1974, she heard that the child of a friend in nearby East Haddam was having a prolonged illness with a rash and painful joints. On June 20 of the next year Polly's son, Todd, had a bite around which there developed a ring-shaped rash; subsequently he had widespread tingling and a severe headache. Five days later the father, Gil, had an acute illness, followed a few weeks later by two enlarging red rings on his back, symptoms that recurred throughout the summer. At that stage Polly was convinced that her family's problems were due to an unknown infectious agent. By August two of her children, Todd and Sandy, were on crutches with painful, swollen knees. Todd's pain continued, and during the following month he was diagnosed as having juvenile rheumatoid arthritis.

Polly learned of other affected children in East Haddam, two living next door to each other, and she discovered four more cases in Lyme. Another mother, Judith Mensch, had a daughter who in the summer of

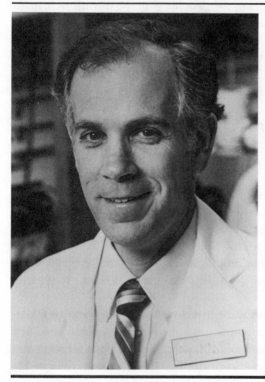

Allen Steere. Now Professor of Medicine at Tufts University School of Medicine, Steere played the leading role in elucidating Lyme disease.

1975 was also diagnosed as having juvenile rheumatoid arthritis. Several other neighbors were similarly affected.

In October 1975 Mrs. Murray telephoned the Department of Health Services and spoke to an epidemiologist, David Snydman. She suggested that an infection might be responsible for the disease. At about the same time, Mrs. Mensch spoke to the State Health Department and to the Centers for Disease Control. It was the combination of the two independent calls that gave extra impetus to the subsequent inquiry. During the next few weeks, Polly conducted a campaign by telephone and by word of mouth. In all, she identified forty-seven cases with similar symptoms.

Snydman knew Allen Steere from their days together at the Centers for Disease Control. But by 1975 Steere had moved to the Yale University School of Medicine to begin a rheumatology fellowship under the direction of Stephen Malawista. Snydman contacted Steere and asked if he would be willing to investigate this apparent clustering of arthritis cases. So it was that Polly Murray and Judith Mensch both went to the Yale clinic to meet Steere.

Steere and his colleagues had no difficulty establishing that there had been an epidemic. In three local townships, with a total population of twelve thousand, a similar arthritis had developed in thirty-nine children and in twelve adults during the past four years. Half of the patients lived on only four streets.

There were other clues. Most of the victims lived in heavily wooded areas; the onset of their illness was usually in the summer months, between June and September. The disease sometimes began with fever and flu-like symptoms. A quarter of the patients reported a peculiar red rash that gradually expanded over a considerable area. This rash was usually on the chest, abdomen, back, or buttocks rather than on exposed parts, suggesting a bite by a crawling insect rather than a flying insect. The arthritis consisted of brief attacks of swelling in a few large joints over a period of several years. Steere's initial conclusion was that this was a previously unknown disease, probably caused by a crawling insect. Only after ongoing study of patients with the typical rash did it become apparent that it was a more general illness sometimes associated with the nervous system or the heart.

When the skin department at Yale was consulted, it happened that a young physician from Denmark was present. He explained that a similar rash was known in Scandinavia. In 1909 a Swedish physician, Arvid Afzelius, had described such a rash following a bite by an insect, but in Europe no arthritis was reported. The Scandinavians had shown that the tick was *Ixodes ricinus*. In 1913 an Austrian physician called the rash erythema chronicum migrans, meaning a chronic, migrating red rash.

By 1977 nine patients in the neighborhood of Lyme remembered having been bitten by a tick. One tick was saved. A dark brown insect the size of a pinhead, it could be easily overlooked. Biologists at Yale set animal traps and established that the tick was exceptionally common in the immediate vicinity of the arthritis epidemic. Two years later Andrew Spielman at Harvard decided that the tick belonged to a different species and named it *Ixodes dammini*. It was a close relative of the tick that had been described by the Scandinavians as the cause of a rash in humans.

As expected, the ticks were not confined to Lyme but were spread by local animals. In 1981 ticks were collected from the woods on Long Island, about twenty miles away, as part of the routine surveillance for Rocky Mountain fever. These ticks were sent to Willy Burgdorfer, an international authority on tick-borne disease working in Montana. To his surprise, the intestine of one tick contained large numbers of spirochete bacteria, similar in appearance to those that cause syphilis but unrelated to that illness and completely different in effect.

Burgdorfer's spirochete was grown in culture, which made it possible to study the stored blood of patients afflicted with what, by then, was called Lyme disease. This work demonstrated that the patients had developed specific antibodies against that particular organism. Experts at the University of Minnesota Medical School used sophisticated tests on the organism and proved that it was an unknown species in the genus *Borrelia*. In 1984 it was named after its discoverer, *Borrelia burgdorferi*.

This *Borrelia* was subsequently identified in deer, voles, field mice, and migratory birds. It is also believed to cause disease in horses and dogs. The organism is present in 20 to 85 percent of the ticks on the North Atlantic coastline of the United States, and in only 3 percent of ticks on the West Coast, which would explain, in part, the original distribution of Lyme disease. Patients with Lyme disease are now being reported throughout the world, particularly in European countries where hiking in wooded areas is a common activity.

Once the causative organism had been identified, it was important to determine whether *Borrelia burgdorferi* reached the synovium in affected joints. Early studies of synovium using modern techniques failed; only after resorting to older techniques were spirochetes occasionally visible under the microscope. As with reactive arthritis, this painstaking work is seldom successful. So far, it has been impossible to identify more than a single spirochete in a specimen. The organism could be alive in the synovium, for it has been grown in cultures of synovial fluid. But this has happened only twice in fifty attempts.

The most encouraging aspect of this intriguing story is that it has led to methods of prevention and treatment. It is impossible to eradicate the reservoir of ticks in wild animals and birds, but humans can adopt preventive measures by wearing suitable clothes and reducing exposure to ticks wherever they are prevalent. Throughout the United States are notices warning of the dangers of ticks. As for treatment of *Borrelia burgdorferi* infection, penicillin is effective in most cases if the course is started early enough.

Thus, there are similarities and differences among the arthritis of Lyme disease and the reactive arthritis following sexually acquired infection or dysentery. In all three we find clear evidence of infection, disease transmission, epidemics, and antibodies formed against certain microorganisms; and, at least with Lyme disease and dysentery, bacteria are accepted as the cause. Clinical observations of Lyme disease, including its spread through the body, the recurrent arthritis over several years, and the nature of the organism, all suggest that the arthritis is often due to continuing infection with live organisms. By contrast, the clinical findings in reactive arthritis are consistent with the view that the arthritis is a reaction to dead bacteria.

In due course, studies of synovium and synovial fluid from people with Lyme disease will be conclusive, but so far the results are difficult to interpret. In the majority of samples taken from joints, bacteria have not been found; two positive cultures are by no means decisive. There remains the possibility that, in the arthritis of Lyme disease, a reaction to dead bacteria is sometimes an important mechanism, as in reactive arthritis.

6

Access to the Joints

As Sir Arthur Conan Doyle was a physician, it is not surprising that he created Sherlock Holmes as the ideal solver of challenging problems. It was a decision that causes embarrassment to both physicians and detectives, because Holmes was always right and therefore set a standard that is impossible to follow. Were his problem discovering the causes of arthritis, there is no doubt that Holmes would have taken the first opportunity to study how foreign substances gain access to the body and to the joints. Next, he would have concentrated on the conundrum posed by the fact that foreign substances can act as antigens and cause arthritis, yet escape detection during an investigation of the synovium and synovial fluid using the best modern techniques. How, then, does a foreign substance gain access to the body and to the joints? This is an aspect of arthritis research that has been relatively neglected by rheumatologists until recent years.

In 1924 Ludwig Aschoff, Professor of Pathologic Anatomy at the University of Freiberg in Germany, reviewed the whole subject of how cells assist in the body's defenses. It was a field in which he had been one of the main contributors. After Metchnikoff's discovery of the phagocytic property of macrophages, polymorphs, and other cells, it was shown that virtually all cells have the ability to engulf foreign substances under certain circumstances. This knowledge was of immense benefit at about the turn of the century because many cells had been identified without knowing what they did or how to classify them. One approach, adopted by many experimental pathologists, was to perform dynamic studies after supplying live cells with dyes such as lithium carmine, pyrrhol blue, and trypan blue, and minute particles such as those of carbon. The researchers could then follow the cells to determine what they did and how they were distributed in the body. This technique gained impetus from Ehrlich's introduction of the use of dyes in chemotherapy, starting with Salvarsan.

Investigators gradually gathered a vast amount of information. For instance, dyes injected into the skin of animals were found in cells in the lymph nodes, spleen, liver, lungs, blood vessel linings, nerves, adrenal glands, and pituitary gland. But it was not until 1911 that Aschoff saw the central theme in all that had been learned. He concentrated on the "reticuloendothelial cells" of the lymph nodes, spleen, liver, and bone marrow as the most active in this process, and coined the collective name "the reticuloendothelial system." It represented a highly efficient, lively arrangement for removing foreign particles from the blood and lymph vessels. Years before, in 1860, Virchow had reached the more limited conclusion that lymph nodes act as barriers and strain off foreign material brought to them in lymph vessels.

Let us look now at the efficiency of the body's protection against potential antigens in the environment. In this we are not concerned with fluids and soluble substances, which gain entry to the body and to the joints without difficulty. This ready entry of fluids and soluble substances applies not only to the stomach and intestines, but also, for instance, to the lungs. Inhaled anesthetics and tobacco products have no trouble getting into the bloodstream and reaching the brain and many other organs. From the standpoint of arthritis, our interest is in larger molecules and particles, such as proteins and silica.

Substances painted on the skin are soon ingested by phagocytic cells under the skin, and from there they are quickly conveyed via local lymph vessels to lymph nodes. In a similar way carbon, silica, and asbestos particles that enter the lungs are taken up by phagocytic cells and removed by either lymph or blood vessels. Unfortunately, in both instances the researchers who reported this work did not determine what happened after that, or whether the substances they were studying entered the main circulation or the joints.

The intestines are filled with a large mass of antigenic material. To protect us from this material, we have a complicated physical barrier and a specialized component of the immune system. Nevertheless, foreign proteins undoubtedly do get through. The intestinal wall is extremely efficient, but far from perfect. Many of the substances that pass through are destroyed in the liver, but a proportion evade the liver by going up a large specialized vessel (the thoracic duct) and entering the bloodstream intact.

In summary, we delude ourselves if we think that we have complete protection from the antigens that surround us. There is always a small proportion of foreign substances in our bloodstream.

We are sadly ignorant about how foreign substances are transported. Perhaps the reason is that scientific interest has focused predominantly on infections by live organisms, rather than on the stray antigens that cause arthritis. In general terms, we know that some substances are conveyed independently in the bloodstream and that some are transported within cells. But we do not know which of these methods applies to substances that enter the joints. Certain bacteria are usually transported in cells to other sites in the body. This applies to several bacteria known to be closely associated with joint disease (mycobacteria, chlamydia, salmonella, yersinia, gonococci).

Antigens destined for the joints are almost certainly transported both independently and in cells, but let us assume for the present that transport within cells is the more important mechanism. By this method certain cells would engulf the antigens at the portal of entry and then convey them to the joints. Many cells would be destroyed in the lymph nodes and the rest of the reticuloendothelial system, but some cells would enter the blood vessels in the joints—in sufficient numbers to cause arthritis.

Cohnheim made an immense contribution to rheumatology, and to medicine as a whole, when he established that in inflammation cells are recruited in large numbers from distant parts of the body. He also showed that when the cells reach the local area in the bloodstream, they pass through the lining of small blood vessels into the tissues. It was recognized at the time that gaps exist between the cells lining the blood vessels, and that these gaps become larger in inflammation. Knowledge has progressed since then.

The first event in inflammation is the dilation of the smallest blood vessels. In some vessels that ordinarily carry little blood, a steady flow develops. The blood in the smallest veins (venules) divides into separate streams, with only plasma near the vessel lining. The rate of blood flow diminishes: the white blood cells move to the periphery, and some begin to stick to the lining of the vessel. At first, most cells tend not to stick and get washed away. Then, numerous cells adhere to the vessel lining and roll along it. Finally, the rolling cells move to the junctions between the endothelial cells and migrate through these gaps into the surrounding tissues. Figure 11 shows in diagrammatic form cells, proteins, and particles passing through the lining of a small blood vessel.

For those in arthritis research, two of the most important questions are how those cells become adherent, and how they get through the vessel lining into the joint. The lining of the small veins (venules) is the final barrier between the world outside and the joint; and a supply of antigens is in the bloodstream, ready to enter.

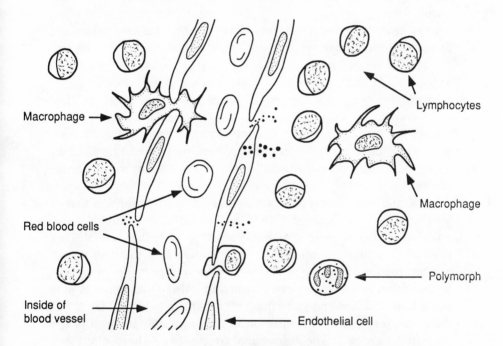

Figure 11 • Cells, proteins, and particles pass through the lining of a small blood vessel. In the bloodstream are red cells, which are disc shaped. In the tissue around the blood vessel are several lymphocytes with round nuclei, also a large cell (macrophage) and a smaller cell with three lobes (polymorph). Passing through the blood vessel wall are a macrophage, a lymphocyte, and different-sized proteins and particles.

Within the past few years, the function of the endothelial cells lining blood vessels has become a major focus of investigation. At last it has been fully appreciated that endothelial cells play a critical role in initiating and maintaining inflammation. These cells have many dynamic functions, including the processing and presentation of antigens. They also have numerous receptors and signaling mechanisms that, among other functions, control the homing of macrophages and lymphocytes, provide molecules that ensure adherence of appropriate cells within the bloodstream, and promote their passage through the venular lining into the tissue.

When considering the role of the venular lining as a barrier, we need to bear in mind that its functions under normal circumstances become markedly aggravated at times of inflammation. Then the gaps between the lining cells are wide open and cells pour into the tissues: the barrier is truly down.

Damage to the blood vessels may be permanent. One great advantage to studying the human eye is that it has a window through which you can see the vessels in the retina at the back of the eye, as well as the leakage of any fluid or cells from those vessels. It is well known to ophthalmologists that once the retinal vessels have been inflamed, they never recover completely. In addition, experimental evidence shows that the same principle applies to vessels in joints. Once a joint has been persistently inflamed, in theory it may become prone to invasion by many more antigens—to the point where it is no longer an effective barrier.

The first successful experiments using dyes to study the function of joint vessels were conducted in 1936 by John Kuhns and Harold Weatherford of the Department of Anatomy at Harvard Medical School. They injected dyes under animals' skin and showed that the dyes readily reached the joints via the bloodstream. The transported material was found within macrophages in the synovium. Also, large amounts were in the bone marrow and small quantities in the muscles and fat. When there was preexisting inflammation in the joints, the amounts of dye deposited increased. The researchers concluded, without direct evidence, that inert substances injected into the skin might be conveyed through the bloodstream within phagocytic cells, and that the same mechanism might transport other materials, including bacterial and metabolic (food) products. In 1939 two other workers provided more detailed evidence concerning the passage of proteins and bacteria into the synovium. Then came World War II, as well as the official rejection of the concept of focal sepsis. Whatever the reason, this promising line of research was not pursued for another thirty years; it has not yet been taken to its logical conclusion.

Which parts of the joint are most vulnerable to invasion by foreign substances? Infection of human joints by live bacteria, particularly the tubercle bacillus discovered by Koch, provides a good model. In children, joint infection by tubercle bacilli (and other bacteria) often results from organisms in the blood being deposited first in the bone marrow near the joint. The consequence is a local focus of infection within the bone, which only secondarily spreads to the synovium and the rest of the joint. Adults also have joint infection as the result of tubercle bacilli carried in the bloodstream, but in them the infection more frequently begins in the synovium.

The fact that bacteria may be deposited in either the bone or the synovium corresponds well with the findings of Kuhns and Weatherford. There is another reason for thinking that bone marrow, which has always been regarded as a more orthodox member of the reticuloendothelial system than the synovium, may be particularly vulnerable: its circulation is different. Because blood is formed in bone marrow, there are not the usual capillaries and venules. Instead, the small arteries open into lakes of blood, which are drained by small veins (similar to the arrangement in lymph nodes). This type of anatomy lends itself to the deposition of foreign substances. Particles in the bloodstream, besides being deposited in the synovium and the bone marrow, may also be deposited in the outer lining of the bone (periosteum) and in the tissues that surround the joint capsule. Figure 12 depicts foreign particles where they may be deposited: in synovium, in bone, and in periosteum. It is worth noting that arthroscopy permits investigation of synovium and synovial fluid, but not of bone or periosteum.

The prolonged failure to find organisms in the joints of people with common types of arthritis understandably led to the false impression that a joint is a protected site into which nothing can enter. Instead, we can now reach four conclusions. First, a joint is vulnerable to invasion by foreign substances and to some extent can be regarded as part of the reticuloendothelial system. Second, in response to this invasion, a joint can respond in a manner similar to the reaction of a lymph node to the wide variety of substances that enter it. Third, once a joint becomes inflamed, the entry of foreign substances increases markedly. Fourth, fol-

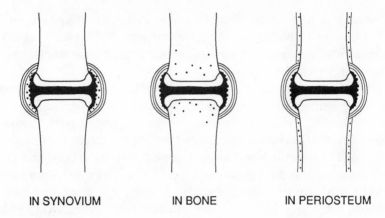

IN SYNOVIUM   IN BONE   IN PERIOSTEUM

Figure 12 · Foreign particles may be deposited in synovium, in bone, and in periosteum.

lowing a persistent episode of inflammation of a joint, functional or structural changes in small blood vessels may make that joint far more vulnerable to invasion by many different substances.

Toward the end of the nineteenth century, microbiologists accepted the concept that some forms of infection were probably caused by organisms other than bacteria, but they were wrong in thinking that it was just a matter of time before they could grow all such organisms in culture. They did not appreciate that there might be viruses—organisms that could not thrive except as parasites within cells.

The word "virus" is a chameleon. Throughout the centuries it has regularly changed its meaning and may continue to do so. Its original Latin meaning was "slime," but by the time of Christ it meant "poison" or, occasionally, "odor" or "sharp taste." By the seventeenth century, reflecting the ignorance at the time, the word was used in England to mean any poison or other substance that might cause an infection, without implying the presence of microbes. In the early part of the nineteenth century, before the germ theory was proved to be correct, the word "virus" meant either a chemical poison or a microbe. After 1876 poison was dropped from the meaning, and the word included all types of microbes.

It is a popular belief that in science the person who first stumbles on a new observation and initiates a breakthrough is necessarily the person who deserves the most credit. But, as Paul Ehrlich often remarked, what matters in research is not the initial discovery, it is what one thinks and does next. The first identification of viruses makes this point, following as it does the pattern of many discoveries in the history of science. Two men made observations that handed them the opportunity to make a famous advance, but they failed to perceive what Nature had offered them.

In 1879 Adolf Mayer, a German chemist, began to study tobacco mosaic disease because it was destroying the tobacco crops in the Netherlands. He proved that the disease was infectious by inoculating healthy plants with the sap from diseased plants. Then, having failed to culture any organism, he passed the infectious sap through a simple paper filter and showed that the filtered fluid was still infectious. After further experiments he concluded, "The mosaic disease of tobacco is a bacterial disease, of which, however, the infectious forms are not isolated nor are their form and mode of life known."

A Russian student, Dimitri Ivanowski, learned of Mayer's work and spent three summers doing research on tobacco plantations, reaching no useful conclusions at that time. He then learned of the discovery of diphtheria toxin and concluded that the filtered sap might have contained a bacterial toxin. To test this hypothesis, he passed the sap through a filter known to remove bacteria and found that the filtered material was still infectious. This did not surprise him because he was looking for a toxin and, so far as he was concerned, that was what he had found. His only alternative explanation, until the work of Martinus Beijerinck had been published, was that the filter might have failed to remove some bacteria.

Martinus Beijerinck (1851–1931) was born in Amsterdam, the son of a tobacconist. With the financial help of his uncle, he studied chemistry at Delft Polytechnic. There he was stimulated intellectually by his roommate and close friend, Jacobus van't Hoff, who in 1901 won the Nobel Prize in chemistry for establishing the laws of osmosis. Later Beijerinck attended a three-year course in botany in Leiden. After an unhappy period working for a commercial firm, in 1895 he was appointed Professor of General Microbiology at Delft, where he directed a new microbiology laboratory.

Beijerinck first worked on tobacco mosaic disease in 1879, at the suggestion of Adolf Mayer. Having no experience in microbiology, he made no progress and temporarily abandoned the problem. He did not return

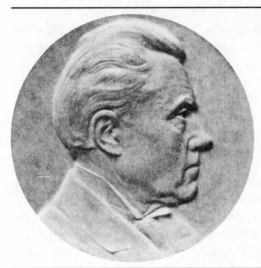

Martinus Beijerinck. Working in Delft, Beijerinck established the modern concept of viruses when he demonstrated organisms that are not cellular and can reproduce themselves only within host cells.

to it until 1897, when he had his own microbiology laboratory. He then took the logical steps that Mayer and Ivanowski had failed to take. First, he demonstrated that the disease could be transmitted through an un-limited succession of plants, from which he concluded that what was being transferred must be alive and capable of multiplying itself—and therefore not a toxin. He then placed a sample of sap on a solidified culture medium of agar. Some time later he noted that the sap on the surface of the culture medium was still infectious. More important, he scraped some agar from just below the surface and found that it too had become infectious, thus indicating that the infectious material could dif-fuse like a liquid. If the organism passed through a filter and could dif-fuse like a liquid, it could not be composed of cells. He concluded that he was investigating an organism that could reproduce itself and yet was not cellular, in direct opposition to Virchow's dogmatic statement that everything alive and capable of reproduction must be cellular. This con-ceptual leap required immense courage. Furthermore, Beijerinck knew that the organism could reproduce itself only in the plant, not outside it. His next proposal was made in the full awareness that it was contrary to Nature: he suggested that, in order to reproduce, the organism incorpo-rated itself into the cells of the plant. We now know that Beijerinck was correct in proposing that a virus is obliged to live and reproduce as a parasite within cells.

It is not surprising that scientists were slow to adopt Beijerinck's concept of an organism that was not cellular and could reproduce itself only within the cells of a host. Half a century elapsed before the structure of viruses was studied with the electron microscope and Beijerinck was vindicated at last. Later, viruses were investigated in detail and are now characterized by their core of DNA (deoxyribonucleic acid) or RNA (ribonucleic acid).

Arthritis may be caused by either acute or persistent viral infections. Well-known examples of acute viral arthritis include those associated with German measles (rubella), hepatitis, parvovirus, mumps, and the Ross River virus of Australia. All of them have similar clinical features.

Rubella is a worldwide disease in children and young adults. When it presents in an obvious form, it is characterized by fever, a faint rash on the trunk, and enlarged lymph nodes at the back of the neck. Often, though, it is so mild as to escape detection, and the illness lasts for only a few days. Because it is such a mild complaint, rubella attracted little attention until it was found that it could lead to congenital deformity. Since the introduction of vaccination it has become much less common.

Rubella arthritis was first described in 1906 by William (later Sir William) Osler (1849–1919). Born in Ontario, he graduated from McGill University in Montreal in 1872. He became a professor at McGill, at the University of Pennsylvania, and then at the Johns Hopkins University before moving to Oxford University as Regius Professor of Medicine. The outstanding physician of his time, he had an immense influence on medicine and medical education in all three countries; this remained particularly true in my own medical school at McGill.

The arthritis of rubella is an acute condition involving many joints, occurring predominantly in girls and young women. It begins at approximately the same time as the rash, when the virus is present in the blood. As with all types of acute viral arthritis, it is difficult to diagnose the cause of the arthritis when it is accompanied by little if any other clinical evidence of disease. Usually the arthritis subsides completely within a week, but in rare instances it may persist for months. After the illness has disappeared, rubella virus, like several other viruses, can remain in the blood for years without causing any harm. Some researchers have suggested that persistent rubella virus may be important in the causation of rheumatoid arthritis, but the evidence is slender.

Until recent years the most familiar examples of persistent viral infections were mouth and genital herpes. In both types the virus remains localized for the rest of the individual's life. Most of the time it lies dormant in nerve cells within the head or within the pelvis, until it is provoked by stress or some other stimulus that induces it to emerge intermittently and cause clinical evidence of infection. On rare occasions, episodes of clinical herpes are associated with recurrent attacks of acute arthritis, usually confined to a few joints and lasting only about a week. Recent evidence suggests that these attacks may be due to a specific defect in the immune system.

The appalling worldwide epidemic of AIDS today is familiar to everyone. In Africa alone, millions of people will die of this disease. In Kampala, the capital of Uganda, the prevalence of positive blood tests among pregnant women and unselected blood donors in 1989 was over 20 percent. To quote the *New England Journal of Medicine:* "Old and young, men and women, rich and poor, rural and urban, married and single are all commonly infected. Similarly, members of all ethnic groups, religions, and professions are at risk."

In contrast to such tragic devastation, arthritis does not kill, but it does have a significant effect on the quality of life and it presents many problems for physicians in diagnosis and management. In New York, between 1981 and 1986, fourteen patients with florid arthritis at the Hospital for Joint Diseases were investigated in the department directed by Robert Winchester. All of these patients were found to have AIDS, and in several of them the arthritis was the first evidence of that disease. Since then, similar patients have been seen throughout the world. The most frequent presentation is with sexually acquired reactive arthritis, and that is what Winchester and his colleagues described. Later reports included psoriatic arthritis, polymyositis (inflamed muscles), Sjögren's syndrome (swollen glands with dry eyes and mouth), and infection of bones and joints by live organisms.

From 1985 to 1989 my colleagues Ian Rowe and Andrew Keat played leading roles in a collaborative study conducted at St. Stephen's, St. Mary's, and Westminster Hospitals in London. At that time approximately 2,750 individuals were attending those hospitals because they had positive blood tests for the human immunodeficiency (HIV) virus. The medical group at the hospitals located 123 patients with rheumatic complaints, all but 4 of whom were men. Thirty-six patients had an inflammatory arthritis that resembled reactive arthritis; 13 had inflamed

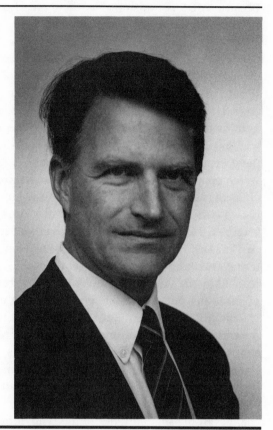

Robert Winchester. Currently at the College of Physicians and Surgeons in New York, Winchester described the association between arthritis and AIDS, and established the molecular basis for inherited susceptibility to rheumatoid arthritis.

muscles; 23 had spinal pain; and 9 had infections of the bones or joints. The remainder had a variety of disorders that were harder to classify. This mixture of types of joint disease is already causing many diagnostic difficulties; such problems are certain to increase as the full force of the AIDS epidemic is felt.

One crucial issue is early diagnosis. In London approximately half of the patients present with rheumatic symptoms at a time when HIV infection has not been confirmed. When there is arthritis of uncertain cause in a young man, it is essential to review the risk factors for AIDS, but it is not yet considered ethical to do the appropriate blood test without obtaining permission after a full explanation. Accordingly, the test may not be done when AIDS seems no more than a remote possibility.

Because AIDS is transmissible, there are also difficulties in performing invasive procedures such as arthroscopy.

The reactive arthritis associated with AIDS attracts considerable attention. Quite apart from AIDS, sexually active homosexual men are at greater risk of developing reactive arthritis than most other groups in society, so it is not certain whether AIDS actually predisposes to reactive arthritis. The early impression is that it does, and that it also makes the arthritis more severe than expected. But these hypotheses are going to be difficult to prove. Forward-looking studies are being organized, but there are obvious problems in arranging a formal research project in which people with similar life-styles are selected to act as controls.

There is also appreciable interest in the immune response in AIDS. It is a characteristic of the disease that the virus destroys a certain type of T-cells (CD4 cells). It has been argued that because reactive arthritis occurs in AIDS, the CD4 cells may not play an active role in reactive arthritis without AIDS. Another proposal is that the immune defect (caused by the virus) makes people susceptible not only to a wide range of infections, but also to different types of arthritis.

In addition, it is theoretically possible that the virus may also damage the endothelial lining of small blood vessels. My colleagues at Westminster Hospital, led by Nigel Harcourt-Webster, recently reported a large series in which they had studied joints of people with AIDS at postmortem. Although none of these people had had joint symptoms, the majority, even those with disease of short duration, showed remarkable changes in the small arteries of the synovium. There is no evidence yet that damage to the endothelial cells enables other organisms to enter the joints.

It is a common misconception that—apart from brief invasions by bacteria or viruses during an illness—microorganisms rarely penetrate the skin, the intestinal wall, and the other physical barriers that protect us from the environment. Perhaps it is more reassuring to pretend to ourselves that our bodies are immaculately clean, while recognizing in our more perceptive moments that this cannot be true. In reality, many organisms live successfully inside us, usually causing no symptoms and sometimes surviving for the rest of our lives. Furthermore, remnants of dead bacteria are always present. Indeed, the constant stimulus of this microscopic material may be as essential to our well-being as vitamins.

A second misconception, common among doctors and scientists, is that if these foreign organisms and substances do not cause the customary clinical features of infection, they are probably not important. As we shall see later, this assumption is incorrect insofar as joints and arthritis are concerned.

There is a third misconception. Although most people find the subject distasteful, we must raise it as a possible cause of arthritis in many millions of people. Sitting in the comfort of our homes in America, Europe, or Australia, it is all too easy to forget about parasites—another confusing, multipurpose word. By definition, a parasite is any organism that lives on (or in) another organism, at the expense of the latter. In theory, this definition includes all types of small organisms; but by tradition the medical study of parasites has been confined to three groups: unicellular organisms called protozoa, worms, and arthropods (the largest group of invertebrates, including insects). The physical structures of medical parasites are complicated; so parasites constitute extremely challenging invaders for our body defenses to overcome because they present to the immune system a wide, and sometimes changing, variety of foreign substances (antigens). Moreover, many parasites have elaborate life cycles, during which these organisms are often transmitted from animals to humans.

Although medical parasites are more common in tropical areas, they infect many people in temperate climates. The number of people infected by parasites is measured in billions; and individuals often have several different parasites. One parasitic worm alone inhabits a third of the human race. When we talk about the disease schistosomiasis, we are referring to about 200 million people with the disease. And when we talk about filariasis, we mean 300 million people.

Given the scale of the problem, and the supposition that many millions of individuals may have arthritis related to parasite infection, one might expect that the main issues would have been thoroughly investigated by now. Sadly, that is not so. We do know, from epidemiological studies conducted several years ago, that much of the arthritis in tropical countries has many of the clinical characteristics of reactive arthritis, thereby suggesting that it may result from infection. When I reviewed the medical literature on this subject, however, I was struck by the lack of detailed information. Even now, it is unusual for there to be any mention of arthritis in standard textbooks on tropical medicine or in specialized monographs on individual diseases such as schistosomiasis.

Even though several people have contributed to the recognition of parasite arthritis, Paul Doury deserves special mention. A Frenchman who spent much of his early professional life working in Africa, he became familiar with tropical infectious diseases, including parasite diseases. On returning to an academic career in Paris, he was consulted by several patients who had lived abroad and now had various forms of arthritis that he attributed to parasite infections. In particular, they recovered from their arthritis after treatment with antiparasite drugs. Doury published his findings and helped to air this important problem. He also drew up and published strict criteria for the diagnosis of parasite arthritis; and he arranged for the postgraduate education of several doctors from countries where parasite arthritis is common.

We now know that a wide range of parasites is associated with arthritis. Sometimes live parasites find their way into the joints or into the tissues around the joints, or the parasites may predispose to secondary bacterial infection. Although the ultimate evidence is not yet available, the likely explanation of most examples of parasite arthritis is that they represent a reaction to fragments of dead parasites, that is, they are forms of reactive arthritis. Yet one apparent difference between parasite arthritis and reactive arthritis following bacterial infection is that parasite arthritis responds more satisfactorily to treatments that destroy the causative organism—in this case, the parasite.

The disease schistosomiasis, as it is seen in Egypt, epitomizes many of the issues related to arthritis associated with parasite infection. The organism that causes this common ailment is a flatworm (or fluke). During its life cycle it reproduces first in humans and then in snails, reinfecting humans by direct penetration of the skin when the individual is standing in water that contains snails. Having penetrated the skin of a human, the young organisms migrate to the lungs and to the ducts of the liver, where they mature and mate. Afterward they pass to the blood vessels in the walls of the intestine and of the bladder. Most people who harbor these worms never have any symptoms; troublesome illness is confined to those with heavy infestation.

In 1966 Magdi Girges, a surgeon in Tanta, Egypt, wrote a brief report in an English medical journal concerning fifty people who were found to have schistosomiasis and arthritis. Thirty-five patients had bladder symptoms, and fifteen had experienced persistent intestinal symptoms due to schistosomiasis. By definition, arthritis was present in all of them. The joints in these people were not swollen, but there was joint pain, mostly in the knees, ankles, and spine. Thirty-six of the fifty patients recovered completely after antiparasite treatment.

Several years later two rheumatologists, Carson Dick of Newcastle in England and A. El-Ghobarey of Cairo, selected an English medical student, Steven Atkin, to do a more formal study of arthritis related to schistosomiasis. He was taught methods of arthritis assessment in Newcastle, then went to Egypt, where he worked alongside Dick's wife, a former ward sister by then working full-time in arthritis research. As soon as arthritis was found in people with schistosomiasis, Dick went to Egypt himself to confirm the findings.

Atkin examined ninety-six patients with active schistosomiasis infection as they attended a medical clinic a hundred miles from Cairo. The complaint was particularly common there following the construction of the Aswan Dam. The average age of the patients was thirty-one years. Fifty-two were men, forty-four were women. Patients with a fever were deliberately excluded from the investigation.

Only twenty-four of the ninety-six patients did not have joint pain. Arthritis in limb joints was found in sixty-three individuals. Often there was pain and swelling of joints in the hands, wrists, knees, ankles, or feet. The characteristic history was that the arthritis began three to fourteen days after the onset of symptoms of the infection. A few patients were followed for long enough to confirm that the arthritic symptoms usually subsided after treatment of the parasitic infection.

The whole story of the relation between parasites and arthritis and what can be revealed by a simple, clinical investigation implies that this is an enormous issue about which we know far too little. There are understandable explanations for our ignorance that concern priorities, personnel, money, facilities, health-care organization, and communication. And only recently have doctors and scientists native to the badly affected countries been in a position to study in depth the arthritic diseases of their own people.

Partly as the result of the efforts of Doury and many like him, it is now extremely encouraging to go to international conferences and listen to rheumatologists and scientists from many countries, busily engaged in the detailed study of types of arthritis that cause pain and disability in millions of their fellow countrymen. Yet, despite all their efforts, most of the obvious research has not yet been done. It is tantalizing to consider what would be learned if massive financial support and other resources were available in developing countries to study parasite arthritis on the vast scale that has been typical of, say, the bacterial type of reactive arthritis and Lyme arthritis. To plan the research would be simple; the benefits would be immense.

We are left with several unanswered questions. Specifically, how a foreign substance can cause arthritis and not be detected by today's highly sophisticated techniques must await reconsideration in later chapters.

Having examined the causes of inflammation anywhere in the body and reviewed the infectious agents that are known to cause arthritis, we must move on to the central problem in arthritis research, which concerns three common diseases: ankylosing spondylitis, psoriatic arthritis, and rheumatoid arthritis. For a century microbes have been sought for all three, but nothing convincing has been found. It is a situation that demands a new approach. Later we shall consider the difficulties encountered by physicians and surgeons in the past as they attempted to understand this complicated group of diseases.

7

Three Key Diseases

As there are many types of arthritis, it is advisable for investigators to study all varieties and to concentrate on a few—such as ankylosing spondylitis, psoriatic arthritis, and rheumatoid arthritis. When we ultimately know the causes of these key diseases, we will understand most arthritis—and many other common diseases of obscure origin as well. Therefore, I will focus on these three types of arthritis and adopt them as both our principal target and a recurring source of clues. They are especially important because the numbers of people in the world thought to suffer from these complaints are staggering: ankylosing spondylitis, 8 million; psoriatic arthritis, 5 million; rheumatoid arthritis, 50 million.

Confronting our selected target, we meet two major clues, neither of which we can afford to ignore. First, despite approaching their causation in many ways and with sophisticated techniques, we have no agreed evidence that any of the three diseases results from episodes of infection or from the action of specific microorganisms. And, second, they are not simple diseases; they are very complicated—which presents a problem for many people because it is in our nature to want things to be straightforward. But arthritis is complex, just as life is complex and each individual is complex. Every person with arthritis is different: John Smith has John Smith's disease; and Mary Jones has Mary Jones's disease. The complicated nature of these diseases is a valuable clue to what causes them.

*   *   *

Ankylosing spondylitis is essentially three distinct disorders that sometimes occur together in individuals, but more often occur in different people. When they appear in one individual, they usually run separate courses, as independent diseases would do. They also respond differently to therapy, so the treatment of one disease does not influence the course of the others.

In its simplest form the first of the diseases, spondylitis, denotes inflammation of the spine in which, apparently spontaneously, the joints and ligaments anywhere in the spine can become inflamed in a diffuse process. In most countries it occurs in about 0.15 percent of the population, and the usual age of onset is between eighteen and thirty-five years. Men are affected about three times as often as women, and most women have less severe disease. In both sexes the severity of the condition may be slight and taper to almost nothing; many people have only minor symptoms. Most people with spondylitis go through life without being diagnosed.

The description of symptoms by the patient is the cornerstone of early diagnosis. For example, a man may complain of persistent lumbar backache for which there is no obvious cause. Usually the onset has been gradual, although it can be abrupt. He may be particularly uncomfortable upon arising in the morning; there may be pain between the shoulder blades, in the neck, or around the chest. Or he may have discomfort in his legs, particularly the thighs, when standing or walking. X-rays early in the disease may show minor changes in the sacroiliac joints within the pelvis, but these changes may not develop for a year or more.

The second disease, acute anterior uveitis, is an inflammation of the iris. It strikes in short, sharp attacks and affects almost as many people as does spondylitis. Again, the onset is often between eighteen and thirty-five years but is common up to age forty-five. Acute anterior uveitis usually affects people who are perfectly fit; it comes out of the blue, and often causes symptoms in only one eye. The pain is so severe that most sufferers go immediately to a doctor and then to an eye specialist. After three to six weeks the eye recovers, usually permanently, but some patients do have subsequent attacks.

The third disease, peripheral arthritis, is an arthritis of joints that are not in the spine but mainly in the arms and legs. This type of arthritis is about as common as acute anterior uveitis. When the arthritis presents in adults, the hips, knees, ankles, or feet are often painful. Joints in the arms may also be affected, but seldom the finger joints. This type of peripheral arthritis is more frequent in men, and once again the onset is between eighteen and thirty-five years—with one important exception. In children, usually only peripheral joints are affected, though after the age of eighteen these young people often develop evidence of disease in the spine or the eyes.

The most significant feature of this triad of spondylitis, uveitis, and arthritis is the complicated relationship among them. Approximately 25 percent of people with spondylitis suffer uveitis at some time, while the remainder never do, despite being exposed to the same environmental triggers. By contrast, 25 percent of people attending eye specialists with acute anterior uveitis have spondylitis, usually undiagnosed until the uveitis draws attention to that possibility. In a similar way, 25 percent of people with spondylitis also have peripheral arthritis. Looking at the people who present first with this type of peripheral arthritis, we find that about half have a previously undiagnosed inflammation of the spine.

The general pattern of these three diseases, then, is of a 25 percent overlap. The principle here is important in the study of causation. When two or more disorders occur in the same individual and behave like separate disorders, they are said to be associated or to overlap; that is, no disorder is the result of another. By contrast, when one disorder is a consequence of another disorder, it is said to be a complication of that disorder.

We have already learned from Ilmari Paronen that reactive arthritis is related to the triad of spondylitis, uveitis, and peripheral arthritis. The early features of reactive arthritis are completely different, but whether it is sexually acquired or follows dysentery, about five years after the onset of reactive arthritis almost half of the patients will have a clinical picture virtually identical to ankylosing spondylitis. This does not mean, though, that we can infer that what caused the reactive arthritis also caused the ankylosing spondylitis.

Next we come to the skin condition psoriasis and to the arthritis sometimes associated with it. Psoriasis is a chronic skin inflammation. For unknown reasons the skin develops pink patches covered with silvery scales, particularly in places subject to pressure, such as elbows, knees, and scalp. One characteristic is that the patches usually disappear and leave almost-normal skin. The carefully defined criteria for psoriasis have been most useful in distinguishing it from similar skin conditions. It is a common disorder, occurring in obvious form in 1 to 2 percent of the population in most countries, but in Japan and in some black populations it is not so common. Onset is frequently in adolescence or early adult life, but it may be at any age. It occurs with greater frequency in some families.

In the arthritis associated with psoriasis (psoriatic arthritis) we have another instance of overlap—this time between psoriasis, peripheral arthritis, and spondylitis, with the peripheral arthritis now dominating the spondylitis. The peripheral arthritis associated with psoriasis is similar to that seen with spondylitis and rheumatoid arthritis.

Psoriasis and psoriatic arthritis occur equally in men and women (unlike the arthritis with spondylitis, which occurs predominantly in men, or rheumatoid arthritis, which occurs predominantly in women). The age of onset of psoriatic arthritis is more evenly spread from childhood to middle age than is true of the other two diseases; thus, undiagnosed arthritis presenting in early adult life and resembling rheumatoid arthritis raises the possibility of psoriatic arthritis.

One striking difference between the peripheral arthritis of psoriasis and that of ankylosing spondylitis is that the fingers are usually affected in psoriatic arthritis, which is uncommon in spondylitis. This feature makes psoriatic arthritis resemble rheumatoid arthritis, a similarity that requires explanation.

Another feature of psoriatic arthritis is its patchiness—like the skin condition. Also, an odd, asymmetrical distribution of finger joint arthritis is common; both hands seldom have the same joint distribution (unlike rheumatoid arthritis). Sometimes only part of a joint is involved. A further characteristic of psoriatic arthritis is that, like the patches on skin, the arthritis in a certain joint may unexpectedly disappear.

The course of psoriatic arthritis is more unpredictable than that of most other joint diseases. In addition, its special features are well known to doctors, but these are uncommon and occur in only 5 percent of patients. Most of the time psoriatic arthritis looks like rheumatoid arthritis, except to the specialist's eye. That is why the two diseases were not clearly differentiated until recently.

Peripheral arthritis occurs in 7 percent of people with psoriasis, or in 0.1 percent of the entire population. The two conditions behave as separate disorders, starting at different times and varying independently of each other. But exceptions occur when the two disorders begin and worsen at the same time; so they cannot be regarded as totally separate. A more common example would be psoriasis starting at thirteen years of age and arthritis starting at twenty-five years.

Spondylitis with psoriasis is the same as ankylosing spondylitis, apart from minor details. It occurs in one-third of people with psoriatic arthritis. Or, argued the other way, about 20 percent of people with ankylosing spondylitis may have psoriasis at some time in their lives—another association that requires explanation.

It is appropriate to mention here another clinical problem similar to psoriatic arthritis. This is spondylitis associated with chronic inflammation of the bowel, owing to two diseases: ulcerative colitis and Crohn's disease. This is essentially the same as ankylosing spondylitis, and the two bowel diseases are almost as common as spondylitis (occurring in about 1 person in 1,000). Once again, three separate diseases overlap: ulcerative colitis, Crohn's disease, and ankylosing spondylitis. In people with one of the bowel complaints, about 5 to 10 percent have spondylitis, which begins separately and behaves separately. The bowel disorder does not cause the spondylitis, which may begin twenty years before there are symptoms due to bowel inflammation—another strong association we must explain.

— Rheumatoid arthritis is the most common, most damaging, and most important of all types of arthritis. Yet, despite massive research, it remains the least understood joint disease. Rheumatoid arthritis occurs in most countries in 1 percent of the population. Three times as common in women as in men, it may strike at any age—usually between forty and sixty-five years.

The most frequent onset is a slowly progressive, diffuse pain and swelling in the finger joints of middle-aged women, often with painful joints elsewhere, particularly in the feet. At first this condition is difficult to assess because about one-third of all women have intermittent pain and swelling in their hands that do not become more severe. Often the only means of making a firm diagnosis is to keep the patient under observation for several months. Under these circumstances about one-third of those suspected of having rheumatoid arthritis recover spontaneously after a few months and have no further trouble. This tendency to recover is important because it indicates that there are lesser and temporary forms of the disease and suggests that an additional factor leads to the chronicity of arthritis. For the unfortunate few whose disease persists, it may take a year or more before doctor and patient accept the diagnosis of rheumatoid arthritis.

An alternative scenario is that the arthritis begins in any joint, with variable presenting symptoms. The onset may be abrupt and the diagnosis obvious. It is well known that men and women over the age of seventy-five years may have a sudden onset of widespread arthritis that often settles almost as quickly.

The characteristics of rheumatoid arthritis vary so much between individuals that some physicians believe that this type of arthritis may represent several different disease processes. For example, the joints may be swollen and very painful, or very swollen and virtually painless. Or there may be severe pain, serious damage, or gross stiffness with negligible swelling. These features do not necessarily operate in parallel. Whatever the nature of rheumatoid arthritis in an individual, it is usually accompanied by the familiar features of any persistent, widespread inflammation. Marked fatigue and weight loss are common; there may be mild or moderate anemia.

With this confusing disease, it is difficult to know how to classify other features occasionally associated with it. Are they merely associated (in the same sense as uveitis and ankylosing spondylitis), or are they true complications resulting from the effects of the arthritic disease? In rheumatoid arthritis, the inflammation in tendons and muscles indicates that the disease is more diffuse and not confined to the joints. Other conditions, such as nodules in the skin and inflammation of minute blood vessels, probably represent complications, whereas scarring of the lungs, dry eyes and mouth, and scleritis (an inflammation of the white of the eye) are probably associations. None of these conditions is a feature of ankylosing spondylitis or psoriatic arthritis.

Another difference among our three key diseases—rheumatoid factor in the blood—is associated with rheumatoid arthritis but not with ankylosing spondylitis or psoriatic arthritis. In 1937 Erik Waaler of the University of Oslo discovered an unusual protein in the blood of people with rheumatoid arthritis. When he published his results, he did not know what the protein was or what it did, so he noncommittally called it a "factor." Then, as often happens in science, the same protein was rediscovered in New York in 1948, and the new results were published without knowledge of the previous work. "Rheumatoid factor" then dominated all arthritis research for fifteen years or more. Even now it is still in the pending file. So far as its significance in causing or aggravating rheumatoid arthritis is concerned, further work might lift it to a position of importance—or condemn it as a mere by-product of the disease.

In diagnosis, rheumatoid factor may provide an additional marker when it is difficult to distinguish rheumatoid arthritis from ankylosing spondylitis or psoriatic arthritis, neither of which has increased levels of rheumatoid factor. But it is necessary to appreciate that rheumatoid factor is not specific for rheumatoid arthritis. Although 70 percent of people with rheumatoid arthritis have it in their blood, it is also found in 5 percent of the normal population, which means that three-quarters of those with rheumatoid factor have no evidence of arthritis. Rheumatoid factor is also increased in many other forms of chronic inflammation and in several types of infection. There is good evidence that people with rheumatoid arthritis who have large amounts of rheumatoid factor are more likely to do poorly and to develop certain clinical features such as skin nodules and inflammation of minute blood vessels.

As viewed under the microscope, the basic process of arthritis is similar in these three target diseases. Such variations as are seen depend principally on how active the inflammation is at the time. The main differences among these diseases are clinical: age of onset, frequencies between the sexes, distribution of joints affected, their courses, associated features (including rheumatoid factor), and complications.

This complex clinical problem illustrates the fundamental difficulties inherent in the definition and classification of different types of arthritis; inevitably these definitions and classifications must vary according to the purposes for which they are adopted. A physician consulted by a person with pain must use all available knowledge—however obtained—to build up a comprehensive assessment of that person's disease, so advice can be given about diagnosis, prognosis, practical problems, and treatment. It is a process tailored to the individual. By contrast, different criteria are required when comparing large numbers of individuals in research, perhaps investigated in different countries. Under these circumstances it is necessary to assume that diseases such as ankylosing spondylitis, psoriatic arthritis, and rheumatoid arthritis are comparatively simple, discrete entities. Several years ago internationally accepted criteria were adopted for most types of arthritis. These criteria have been invaluable when establishing the distribution of arthritis throughout the world, and when assessing diagnosis, prognosis, and treatment.

The main disadvantages of these definitions are apparent in basic research. When studying the causes of arthritis, we need to regard each component as separate, being only temporarily grouped together for the purposes of definition, and possibly requiring rearrangement in the light of new knowledge. Otherwise original thoughts are stifled by rigid beliefs.

People often ask why, when there were brilliant clinical observers in the past, so much ignorance and confusion persisted until this century, or why so many of the advances in understanding the fundamental basis of arthritis have occurred during the past two decades. So it should prove enlightening to look at physicians and surgeons in centuries past, who worked to establish new facts under difficult circumstances, and then at those in contemporary times, who take advantage of deeper understanding and improved techniques in order to provide better diagnosis, prevention, and treatment for those who suffer from various forms of arthritis.

Since the beginning of civilization, perceptive physicians throughout the world have occasionally made celebrated clinical observations that are still quoted and revered today. We tend to forget all of the bias and confusion that constituted the establishment view against which they had to struggle, and the mistakes and misconceptions that were commonplace. It is tempting to recall the peaks and to ignore the troughs— as if physicians of poor quality did not exist, and as if it were always easy to recognize clinical features in the patients examined. But medicine was never like that.

We have already encountered the descriptions of rheumatic fever by Thomas Sydenham in the seventeenth century, and the account of sexually acquired reactive arthritis by Benjamin Brodie in 1818. From these and other examples, it may seem that knowledge was accumulated in a steady flow that followed a logical sequence. What we must accept is that these men were giants in times when standards of clinical diagnosis and care were frequently appalling. Most physicians before (and during) the nineteenth century were either disinterested in arthritis or unable to diagnose arthritic conditions.

In the seventeenth and eighteenth centuries many of the physicians in London prescribed for patients without seeing them. As students, instead of training in hospitals, they led monastic lives and studied the writings of ancient Greeks and Romans. Some physicians did visit patients and make observations that are remembered today, but it was mainly apothecaries who saw patients, recorded symptoms, and then applied to learned physicians as they sat in coffeehouses for prescriptions, written in Latin, which included purging, bleeding, leeches, and complicated mixtures of drugs. It is little wonder that many diseases, including most types of arthritis, remained unknown and undescribed.

By comparison, the majority of surgeons lacked formal education and few had a university degree. Instead, surgeons had the advantage of a realistic apprenticeship, after which they did much of the practical work with patients by examining and treating them in hospitals. The best surgeons in London came to be highly respected and sought after. So it is not surprising that surgeons made many discoveries and clinical observations about patients that escaped the learned physicians; Brodie's studies are excellent examples.

In London's prestigious teaching hospitals, science in medicine scarcely existed in either clinical practice or undergraduate education. Although Laennec had invented a primitive stethoscope in 1816, until the middle of the nineteenth century blood pressure apparatus and clinical thermometers did not exist. Physicians were almost totally dependent on their clinical senses.

By that time postmortem examinations were being conducted, and much was learned from them that was not apparent from clinical observations alone. But the purpose of these examinations was to determine the cause of death, so joints were rarely opened and very little was learned about arthritis. No chemical, blood, bacteriology, or other laboratories were available to help.

Turning to Paris, we gain a clearer view of the circumstances in which arthritis and other diseases were studied. In a later chapter on the nervous system, we shall consider the work of Jean-Martin Charcot (1825–1893), whose contributions to neurology, psychiatry, and rheumatology made him one of the most impressive clinical investigators in the history of medicine. Charcot's name is inextricably linked with that most remarkable of all hospitals, the Salpêtrière, which he described as the "grand asylum of human misery." Until the sixteenth century an arsenal of gunpowder had been located in a densely populated district of Paris. The local residents, concerned about the risk and the repeated explosions that took place in their midst, petitioned King Louis XIII, who in 1565 arranged for a new arsenal to be built on a 90-acre site on the left bank of the Seine, in the angle between the Seine and *la rivière des Go-*

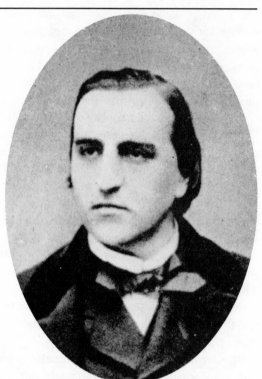

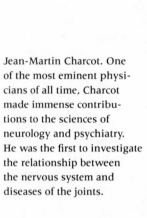

Jean-Martin Charcot. One of the most eminent physicians of all time, Charcot made immense contributions to the sciences of neurology and psychiatry. He was the first to investigate the relationship between the nervous system and diseases of the joints.

belins—outside the city limits. Because of the saltpeter in the gunpowder, this site soon became known as the "Little Arsenal-Salpêtrière."

By royal edict, in 1656 a group of hospitals was created for the confinement of poor beggars, unwanted women, and the infirm; the Salpêtrière was devoted to caring for women and prostitutes. The following year an attempt was made to arrest as many as possible of the fifty-five thousand beggars then believed to live in Paris and to confine them on the same site. For almost two centuries the Salpêtrière was the largest asylum in Europe, housing up to eight thousand people, including "the poor, beggars, cripples, incurables, the aged, children, and insane women." Many were born and died as prisoners in the asylum.

One of Charcot's illustrious successors, Georges Guillain, gave a lurid account of the insane and the incurables:

The hands and feet of the most disturbed patients were bound by chains; their bodies were encased in large iron rings which were riveted to the walls. Here they were left, half naked, to wallow in their own filth and excrement. Food was passed to them through the bars of an iron grill, and so was the straw on which they slept. It was also through this grill that their quarters were cleaned by long rakes. During the winter, the pits below, in which the most disturbed patients were incarcerated, were invaded by rats, which often attacked them. During the morning inspections, it was often found that patients had had their faces and limbs damaged by the vicious bites of the rats.

By the time Charcot was appointed to the staff of the Salpêtrière in 1862, conditions had improved, but they were still deplorable. As Pearce Bailey has written:

> Charcot, leader and administrator at the Salpêtrière, dispelled the chaos created by a mixed and mislabeled population of five thousand displaced and crippled bodies and souls, sensing their true plight and the potential they afforded for research and teaching. He transformed the Salpêtrière from a prison and an asylum of unwanted womanhood into one of the great clinical research centers of the world.

Charcot also introduced an essential innovation. Until his time hospital patients were examined lying in bed, usually on their back, which made it virtually impossible to form any impression of the movements of the limbs or spine. Charcot had the patients conducted to his office, where he could examine them properly.

When Charcot was appointed to the Salpêtrière, he and his colleague Edmé-Felix Vulpian undertook a massive review of all the patients, from which emerged one previously unrecognized disease after another. For example, they assessed all the people with tremors and readily identified people with Parkinson's disease (described in 1817 by a London physician, James Parkinson). They also found a few people with senile tremor. In addition, they discovered several patients with a previously unknown disorder: today we call it multiple sclerosis.

As we look back at the history of the discovery of the medical aspects of arthritis, it is easy—and unfair—to ask, Why did our predecessors fail to see what is so obvious to us? Most present-day patients with arthritis can be diagnosed accurately by physicians listening to their stories and examining them. Laypeople recognize rheumatoid arthritis of the hands at a glance. The simple truth is that all of us are blind to the things that we do not expect to see, even when they are obvious. The same problem applied, until this century, to other disorders such as appendicitis and coronary thrombosis.

The concepts of the ancient Greeks about the role of flowing humors in arthritis, including gout, were proving even less correct by the Middle Ages; the resulting confusion lasted virtually throughout the nineteenth century, until about 1860. As an example of the prevailing medical misconceptions, most forms of inflammatory arthritis were labeled as gout; in 1850 the usual view in England was that arthritis of the wrists, hands, and feet should be called "rheumatic gout"; while arthritis of the shoulders, elbows, and knee joints was "chronic rheumatism"—all hopelessly wrong. Germany and France experienced comparable confusion, despite the presence of outstanding investigators.

Some scholars have suggested that rheumatoid arthritis was rare before 1800. This proposal has stimulated considerable controversy, in which evidence from paintings, books, and medieval skeletons has indicated an absence of illustrations or descriptions of rheumatoid arthritis before that time. The problem is that even though no earlier accounts of rheumatoid arthritis can be found, no one could report a condition he was unable to recognize.

In 1800 the first description of rheumatoid arthritis appeared in the well-known thesis by A. Landré-Beauvais of Paris. And in 1859 Sir Alfred Garrod, a London physician, proposed the unsatisfactory name "rheumatoid arthritis," intending to denote an "inflammatory affection of the joints not unlike rheumatism . . . but differing materially from it." He put several conditions under this wide umbrella, including osteoarthritis and many nonarthritic disorders of individual joints—a limited insight that is now accepted as a peak of excellence during a time of chaos. Throughout the present century the concept of rheumatoid arthritis has been defined and redefined; and it has been rendered more clear-cut by new understanding of the diseases that surround it, some of which were previously classified as being within it. It is by far the most defined and investigated of all the arthritic conditions. Yet not until the first decade of the twentieth century was there wide agreement that a distinction should be made between rheumatoid arthritis (as a form of chronic inflammation) and osteoarthritis (as a form of physical wear of the joints).

In the seventeenth century, at about the same time rheumatic fever was being described and analyzed, the skeleton of someone with severe ankylosing spondylitis was reported. Because ankylosing spondylitis was originally perceived as constituting this type of severe deformity of the spine, the word "ankylosing" (meaning "rigid") was incorporated in its name. How much better it would have been, for patients and for phy-

sicians, if the name had been simply "spondylitis," meaning inflammation of the spine.

Knowledge of the clinical features of ankylosing spondylitis, including
uveitis and arthritis in the limbs, accumulated steadily. The two world
wars provided extensive medical experience of young men with very
early disease. They had typical spinal pain but lacked the classic features
of stiff spines with x-ray abnormalities. The surprising belief then developed in some countries, particularly the United States, that spondylitis
was simply a variant of rheumatoid arthritis; as a result, the name
"rheumatoid spondylitis" occurred regularly in textbooks and medical
journals, even as late as 1975.

Arthritis associated with the skin condition psoriasis was a debatable
concept until 1960. Many believed it to be another variant of rheumatoid arthritis. Only since 1975 has virtually everyone accepted the clinical evidence that psoriatic arthritis is a separate disease.

Despite the astute observations of a few physicians and surgeons, until
this century most founders of the scientific study of joint disorders were
people doing basic research in other subjects—rarely giving a thought to
the possible consequences for arthritis. Orthopedic surgery and pathology were the first specialties (apart from medicine and surgery) to concentrate on effective investigations into arthritis, making important contributions from the beginning of this century. Until approximately 1930,
however, clinical medicine and surgery in developed countries were
dominated by the powerful subjects of general internal medicine and
general surgery, as well as by the continuing need for a general approach
to all patients. Even important clinical specialties such as neurology and
orthopedic surgery could not expand as they should. After 1930 the
medical specialty of rheumatology emerged simultaneously in several
countries. Even then, research was confined principally to clinical observations of people with arthritis and did not tackle the fundamental
causes of joint disorders.

The most helpful early research development was the investigation of
different types of arthritis within communities. From this approach
arose the investigation of populations, families, and races throughout
the world. These studies established the frequencies and characteristics
of diseases everywhere and provided crucial information on the influences of heredity and environment. Without this epidemiological research there would have been no foundation on which others could
build, and little progress could have been made.

It was only after World War II that research into the causes of arthritis began in earnest. Even as late as 1970, clinical rheumatology was surrounded by a pioneering atmosphere and spurred on by a widespread view that the physicians in medical specialties such as rheumatology might not be up to the standards of general internists. It is not surprising that recruitment to clinical rheumatology was difficult during this period.

From about 1975 on, everything changed. In several countries many of the best medical school graduates were keen to enter clinical rheumatology, and many of the best scientists and physicians applied to do basic research into the causes of arthritis. It has been rewarding and exciting to see the world's leading scientists attracted to the enigma of arthritis.

8

The Many Faces
of Arthritis

All four diseases that I have chosen to describe in this chapter are important, though for different reasons. They are polymyalgia rheumatica, Behçet's disease, systemic sclerosis (scleroderma), and systemic lupus erythematosus (SLE).

There are two main reasons why polymyalgia rheumatica must be described in any book about arthritis. First, it is the condition that is most frequently misdiagnosed despite the fact that once you are familiar with it, you can suspect the diagnosis almost as soon as the patient starts to describe the symptoms. Second, it rivals gout as the most treatable of all painful disorders. For the rheumatologist, the diagnosis and treatment of polymyalgia rheumatica is highly rewarding and because almost all patients do well, it is certainly an easy way for a doctor to make friends.

Although polymyalgia rheumatica was recognized during the nineteenth century, it remained obscure until after 1950 and was not given its present name until 1957. When any disease is first recognized as a separate entity, deciding what to call it is always a dilemma. Without an engaging name, it will never command respect and attract attention, but if the cause is unknown, an inappropriate name may prove to be misleading for years to come. In this instance, such problems were avoided by selecting a name almost without meaning. Quite simply, "polymyalgia rheumatica" denotes many painful muscles occurring in a rheumatic disorder.

The disease almost exclusively affects people over fifty-five years of age; the older you are, the more likely you are to develop it. Whereas the frequency in the total population is only about 1 in 2,500, among people over eighty it is twenty-five times as frequent. As a consequence, it is half as common as rheumatoid arthritis in people over seventy years of age. In short, it is a condition of the elderly and therefore is rapidly becoming more frequent in developed countries. It occurs in women twice as often as in men.

One of the characteristic features of polymyalgia rheumatica is that its onset is usually insidious. Sometimes for months, patients assume that their symptoms are due to old age and that they must learn to live with them. They frequently retire from work or give up other cherished responsibilities before seeking medical advice.

At onset there may be only a vague sense of stiffness—little more than is suffered by most people. Then, as the clinical features become more clear-cut, the distribution of pain and stiffness becomes characteristic and is particularly troublesome in both shoulders. Other discomfort may be in the hips, the neck, or the lumbar region. Occasional pain and stiffness occur in the arms and hands, or the knees and other joints; these symptoms lead to some difficulty in distinguishing it from early rheumatoid arthritis. A general sense of stiffness gradually becomes a dominant feature, especially after resting in one place for a length of time. As one cockney sufferer put it, "I am all stiffed up." It is particularly revealing to ask, "If there were a fire in the middle of the night, how quickly could you get out of bed?" To which a common reply is, "I couldn't. I would just have to burn."

Because patients with this complaint often do not consult their doctors, and because the diagnosis is often delayed, polymyalgia rheumatica frequently leads to months of unnecessary pain and disability—or severe disease. I have seen people who, without a diagnosis, were confined to bed in a hospital for months, only to recover completely within days of starting appropriate treatment.

For polymyalgia rheumatica there is virtually only one treatment: a regular, modest dose of a cortisone-like drug, such as prednisone or prednisolone, given by mouth. Despite the current widespread (and unjustified) public prejudice against cortisone-like drugs, there is almost no alternative to this treatment. Symptoms generally improve within hours and often disappear within a week. But recovery may take longer, particularly when the diagnosis has been delayed and the illness is well established. The response to treatment is so dramatic that physicians have a responsibility to prescribe tablets as soon as they suspect the diagnosis.

The patient's response assists considerably in the assessment; if there is no sign of improvement after a week, or tests suggest a different diagnosis, the therapy can be discontinued with no harm done.

With respect to its pathology, polymyalgia rheumatica is a strange condition. It is not primarily an inflammation of the joints, although joints certainly become stiff and occasionally swollen. In about half of untreated people, tests show mild inflammation of medium-sized arteries; but the connection between this and the stiffness of the joints remains unclear.

Apart from the influence of age and the probable association with blood vessel disease, the cause of polymyalgia is not yet known. As with many diseases of unknown cause, it has been suggested that polymyalgia rheumatica may result from a virus infection, but the evidence is thin.

About five years after the onset of polymyalgia rheumatica, approximately one patient in twenty develops true arthritis, with swollen inflamed joints and all the characteristics of rheumatoid arthritis. This suggests two alternatives: either two common diseases are occurring together by chance, or, over time, different causes occasionally lead to classic rheumatoid arthritis.

Behçet's disease is another disorder with a fundamental cause that we do not understand. An unpleasant condition, it may progress in a gradual and often unpredictable manner.

In a previous chapter we discussed an association between eye disease, skin disease, and arthritis. By the beginning of the twentieth century, eye specialists were familiar with Behçet's disease, which is a further example of this association. Then, for many years, eye specialists and skin specialists worked in parallel and wrote separate descriptions of the eye and skin disorders. Several people made the connection between the various features of this complicated condition; but it was not until 1937 that the professor of dermatology at the University of Istanbul, Hulusi Behçet (1889–1948), wrote a description of the disease complex to which his name is attached. Arthritis is common, particularly in the knees, ankles, wrists, and elbows. Additional features are mouth and genital ulcers, and involvement of several other parts of the body. The onset is usually between the ages of twenty and thirty years; and the disease is slightly more common in men than in women.

Of considerable interest is the strange geographic distribution of the disease. It spreads from the eastern Mediterranean to Japan (reminiscent of the Silk Route). The best-documented reports of large numbers of cases have come from Turkey, Iran, China, and Japan. Indeed, it has been estimated that Behçet's disease in Japan is fifteen times as common as in England, and eighty times as common as in Minnesota. The reason for this distribution is unknown. Evidence for a genetic component in families is not strong. At present the only clue to the cause lies in laboratory evidence of an unusual reaction to a common type of virus.

In turning to systemic sclerosis (formerly known as scleroderma), we encounter a disease that is more evenly distributed worldwide and better known. Although uncommon, it teaches us much about the causation of arthritis. The name "systemic sclerosis" is derived from *skleros,* the Greek for "hard." So "scleroderma" denoted the thickening and hardness of the skin, while the new name, "systemic sclerosis," indicates that the hardening is more widespread and affects other organs of the body. The onset of systemic sclerosis is usually in middle life, and it is three times as common in women as in men.

At the time of diagnosis there is often a long history of minor symptoms and physical signs. Because our primary interest is in causes, I concentrate first on the earliest evidence of disease, which relates to small blood vessels. A separate condition called Raynaud's phenomenon, which often precedes systemic sclerosis by several years, usually exists on its own without leading to definite disease, but after several years it may be followed by the onset of systemic sclerosis. Raynaud's phenomenon is essentially a temporary blockage of the circulation in the fingers (or toes), often occurring in attacks precipitated by cold or emotion. The fingers turn white owing to lack of blood, and then they turn blue. As circulation is restored, the vessels dilate and the fingers become red; hence the process is quickly reversible.

In one study of workers who had been exposed to a causative industrial chemical (vinyl chloride, used in the plastics industry), there was clear clinical evidence of systemic sclerosis in 14 percent of those at risk. Microscopic examination of capillaries under the fingernails revealed blood vessel changes in an additional 18 percent. This evidence, coupled with the common relation between systemic sclerosis and Raynaud's phenomenon, suggests that abnormality of the small blood vessels may play a primary role in the development of many of the subsequent clinical features of systemic sclerosis.

The skin disorder, so obvious to our predecessors, prompted the name "scleroderma." These changes are caused by thickening of the skin or by local changes in blood vessels. But thickening of the skin in the fingers can occur in Raynaud's phenomenon alone as the result of altered blood circulation. So to avoid confusion, evidence of more general skin involvement—in the arms, face, or trunk—is required before a diagnosis of systemic sclerosis is made.

Small joints and tendons, particularly in the hands, are commonly affected. Thus, stiffness of the hands in systemic sclerosis often results far more from changes in deep structures and from joint disease than from restriction that results from thickening of the skin. In the joints, the synovium becomes inflamed and most of the other tissues undergo diffuse thickening. Joint damage is seldom severe. In some people the intestines, lungs, heart, kidneys, or muscles may be involved.

Because arthritis is an outstanding feature of systemic sclerosis, we must take seriously the known causes of this uncommon condition, while accepting that they have been identified in only a minority of patients with the disease. In 1914 it was first recognized that there is an increased frequency of systemic sclerosis in miners exposed to silica dust. Since then there have been epidemics related to vinyl chloride and to toxic oil. Other associations are with organic solvents (such as toluene, benzene, and trichlorethylene) and with epoxy resins. Drugs (such as bleomycin and pentazocine) have caused systemic sclerosis, and so has the common (now controversial) practice of enlarging female breasts with paraffin or silicone.

The principal lessons to be learned from systemic sclerosis are twofold. First, damage to small blood vessels can be important in the causation of arthritis; second, the environmental triggers in arthritis may be well beyond the confines of infectious organisms. And what happens in one disease may happen in other similar diseases.

Systemic lupus erythematosus (SLE) is both fascinating and frustrating. For forty years research into the causes of this disease has attracted many of the ablest physicians and scientists. Repeatedly they have seemed to be discovering the answers, only for their work to end in disappointment.

Systemic lupus erythematosus and the subject of autoimmunity go hand in hand. Because autoimmunity is a broad subject of potential importance in several diseases, I will discuss SLE first and then autoimmunity.

The name "systemic lupus erythematosus" has a complicated derivation. "Systemic" implies that the disease may affect many organs and tissues; "lupus" comes from a rare form of the disease that can lead to a facial appearance like a wolf; and "erythematosus" denotes a red rash.

This disease has followed a pattern familiar in medicine. At first it was difficult to diagnose, and only the worst cases were recognized. It is not surprising that these patients fared badly: death was a frequent outcome. Then the ability to diagnose SLE improved dramatically, and people with milder and milder disease were identified. As a result, SLE is now perceived as a common condition that is benign and has a good prognosis. Experience with other diseases has taught us that this pattern of apparent improvement in prognosis can happen without altering the treatment available.

In people with obvious SLE, a general illness is common, with anemia, fever, weight loss, and painful joints and muscles. Psychological problems caused by the disease or involvement of the brain are frequent. Many organs and tissues—skin, kidneys, lungs, heart, eyes, or brain—can be affected in what is truly a systemic disorder.

The joints and tendons are often painful, but swelling is usually mild and permanent damage is rare, in striking contrast to rheumatoid arthritis. Despite similarities in the nature of the persistent inflammation and in the evidence of autoimmunity, in one disease joint damage is rare; in the other, it is common. This contrast may prove to be a valuable clue.

Systemic lupus erythematosus occurs mostly in women younger than forty years of age. Although SLE is eight times as frequent in women as in men, and fifteen times as common during childbearing years, the sex difference does not hold before puberty or after menopause. This striking fact, coupled with a tendency for SLE to begin or become worse during or soon after pregnancy, suggests that sex hormones or sexual maturity may be important factors in causing or modifying the disease.

Reports on the frequency of SLE in different populations vary with the criteria used. In the United States and England the correct figure may be as high as 1 person in 2,000. The disease is more common in blacks in the West Indies and the United States, but curiously it seems much less common in black people in parts of Africa. The frequency of SLE increases about fourfold in Australian aborigines, Japanese, Chinese, and Filipinos. SLE is also more common in the Crow, Arapahoe, and Sioux tribes of North America. A strong genetic component is suggested by the study of SLE in families and in identical twins. It is also common to encounter blood relatives with similar (autoimmune) diseases.

Patients frequently report a history of allergies to drugs and chemicals, long before the onset of their disease. SLE can actually be caused by several drugs, including hydrallazine and procainamide. There are two other clues to the causation of SLE: exposure to sunlight induces marked aggravation of many of the clinical features, and changes in the blood of patients' husbands suggest the possibility of a shared infection.

Now we come to autoimmunity, a difficult subject that has not detached itself completely from its complicated past. Autoimmunity was born at a time when antibodies dominated the subject of immunology. At the end of the nineteenth century there was intense interest in immunity to foreign substances, including bacteria and toxins. Later the immune system was seen to have the capacity to discriminate between self and nonself, so it could protect its own constituent parts while destroying foreign substances that had entered the body. Paul Ehrlich was rightly concerned that if the immune system failed in its ability to discriminate between self and nonself, the consequences would be harmful to the host. How the immune system did or did not react against self was given the ambiguous name of "autoimmunity." Much later the ability of the immune system to live in harmony with self was called "self-tolerance"—a much better and more inclusive name.

I have already mentioned that the Greek belief that diseases were caused by ill-humors was followed by the battle between humoral immunology and cellular immunology. So complete was the victory of the humoralists over the cellularists that Metchnikoff's phagocytic cells and Murphy's lymphocytes suffered remarkable neglect. Antibodies were in the limelight for half a century, after which time some leading immunologists were doubting that immunology had a future.

At the turn of the century it was discovered that antibodies can be formed not only against foreign antigens, but also against constituent parts of one's own body. Ehrlich accepted that these antibodies against self, the "autoantibodies," are formed, but he maintained that some inherent process must prevent them from damaging the individual. One of his theories was that antiantibodies provide a healthy balance between the forces involved—a notion reminiscent of Sir Isaac Newton's third law of motion, which states that action and reaction are always equal and opposite.

Eventually, researchers established that the ability to recognize and tolerate self was learned early in embryonic life. At first this activity in the embryo was thought to be a one-time occurrence, but it soon became accepted that tolerance must continue throughout life—much as Ehrlich had imagined.

With World War I and the death of Ehrlich in 1915, the subject of autoantibodies as possible causes of disease was largely abandoned for several decades. Then, after World War II, it was shown conclusively that antibodies against certain organs cause diseases specific to those organs: for example, thyroiditis, pernicious anemia, and childhood diabetes.

The next problem was almost a recurrence of the humoral-cellular conflict. The consequence has been that some authorities now define an autoimmune disease as "a condition in which damage is produced by the reaction of cells or antibodies with normal components of the body," while for convenience other authorities continue to define autoimmune disease as "disease caused by the action of antibodies against substances normally present in the body." Some immunologists include cells; others do not.

After World War II, when it was established that organ-specific autoimmunity is an important disease process, it was demonstrated that there is also a condition of non–organ-specific autoimmunity. It is essential to emphasize, however, that these two processes are as different from each other as a formal boxing match and an informal free-for-all. In the non–organ-specific form (the free-for-all) it is a question of different antibodies against different organs or parts of the body, which makes it a much more confusing and debatable subject. As an example of this type of autoimmunity, many arthritic diseases (such as SLE, systemic sclerosis, and rheumatoid arthritis) are associated with a wide variety of autoantibodies. In SLE, the premier autoimmune disease in rheumatology, the hallmark of autoimmunity is the presence of antibodies against the nuclear material, DNA; but numerous antibodies also act against other constituents of the body.

It is a popular belief that in an illness such as SLE, the body turns against itself by creating antibodies that damage several organs and tissues. This hypothesis may be partially true—and probably is—but it certainly has not been proved. We do not know why these autoantibodies occur, or how much damage they cause; and there is poor correlation between the number of autoantibodies present and the severity of the disease. As a result, experts cannot agree whether autoantibodies are direct causes of inflammation or simply attractive by-products of the disorder.

Rheumatoid factor is also an autoantibody, and when present in large amounts it is known to be associated with aggravation of rheumatoid arthritis, SLE, and certain other clinical features. But the suggestion that rheumatoid factor plays a central role in the production of disease has never been proved conclusively.

Despite much uncertainty, we do know something about autoimmunity in arthritic diseases. First, there is a genetic component. Family studies of people with autoimmune diseases show a definite increase of autoimmune diseases in close relatives. So it is probable that people are born susceptible to the autoimmune diseases that they suffer later in life.

Since tolerance of self is an ongoing process, it is not surprising that small numbers of autoantibodies and sensitized cells are present in all of us. As Ehrlich predicted, we all have the potential for developing autoimmune diseases, but the vast majority of us are protected by the fine balance between the immune system and self. Because of the sophisticated nature of our heredity and this dynamic equilibrium throughout life, no two patients with autoimmune diseases are exactly alike. Autoimmunity varies with age and from organ to organ. Furthermore, the basic mechanisms may differ fundamentally from one type of autoimmune disease to another.

For decades it has been postulated that autoimmune diseases might be caused by infective agents such as viruses, which lead the body to be confused in distinguishing nonself from self. But as with arthritis in general, years of failure in looking for responsible microorganisms have led many people to believe that foreign substances do not come into play, and that the abnormality generates spontaneously within the individual. In reality, the temporary production of autoantibodies can be induced by several different foreign substances, including drugs, viruses, bacteria, parasites, and food. And the persistent production of autoantibodies can be induced by certain chronic infections. The impression is growing that autoimmunity may superficially resemble hayfever, in which most people have no symptoms but a few inherit an inappropriate reaction to pollens and suffer miserably.

My suspicion is that before long it will be proved that autoimmune diseases are not due to a spontaneous process within the body. Instead, heredity and other factors in the host will be shown to lead to a slightly inappropriate response to many substances that enter the body. How, then, do we explain the autoantibodies, and what are they telling us? It may be that a few of us inherit an immune system that is slightly defective in the way it controls the formation and removal of the autoantibodies we all produce. Disease may result from the testing of the weakened immune system beyond its capacity by one foreign substance or, more likely, by many diverse substances. Thus, foreign substances may be the primary causes of autoimmune diseases, making autoantibodies useful clues—but not major culprits. Whatever the details, depending on the immune systems we each inherit, autoimmune disorders result from a breakdown of the normal controls that enable the body and its defenses to live in harmony.

9

One Gene,
One Disease

Soon after the germ theory of disease was proved to be correct, scientists and physicians questioned whether heredity played a role in susceptibility to infection and to inflammatory diseases of unknown cause, such as arthritis. At first, and for a long time afterward, speculation centered on heredity that appeared to be simple and transmitted by a single gene, now known as Mendelian heredity. So it will be enlightening to consider first the work of Gregor Mendel, then the relevant discoveries in genetics, and, finally, four types of arthritis that follow—or seem to follow—Mendel's laws.

For those unfamiliar with the details of the story, it seems unbelievable that a monk secluded in a monastery during the nineteenth century could be credited with one of the outstanding scientific discoveries of all time. Mendel's father, Anton, was a peasant working on a farm in a village in what is now the center of Czechoslovakia. His son, Johann (later renamed Gregor), was born in 1822. The village community, his father's work, and the farm all were influential in shaping Johann's future. At the village school natural history was deemed to be a particularly important subject. Furthermore, the village priest, a former teacher of natural history, was an expert at grafting fruit trees and kept a small nursery in the presbytery garden. It was he who recognized Johann's abilities and suggested that he be sent away to school.

From then on, Johann's education was paid partly by his parents and partly through his own work. All went well until he was sixteen, when his father had a serious accident that prevented his working any longer

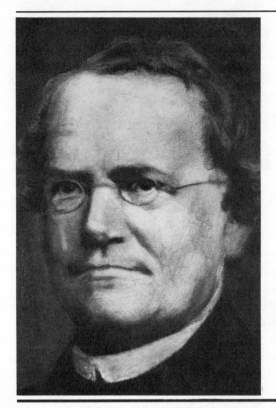

Gregor Mendel. While working in the Brno monastery, Mendel—the father of genetics—showed that discrete particles (later known as genes) convey the messages of heredity.

on the farm. Johann's financial position became so tenuous that he could not have completed his two-year course at Olomouc University if his sister had not renounced part of her dowry to help him.

At the university he studied theology, philosophy, mathematics, physics, and agriculture. When he concluded his studies and was unsure how to continue, his professor of physics helped him to transfer to Brno monastery. Entering as a novitiate, he was renamed Gregor.

For more than forty years Brno monastery had maintained a strong tradition of education and research in natural science. A nursery for the investigation of plant culture had been established in 1825; by the time Mendel joined the monastery in 1843, the type of work that was later to become the basis of his research was already in progress. Also in the monastery were monks who were botanists, mineralogists, philosophers, and mathematicians. It was one of the botanists who taught him how to cross plants in breeding experiments.

At Brno, Mendel studied theology and taught natural science and physics. Because of his outstanding intellectual capacity, the abbot recommended that he be sent to the University of Vienna, where he worked from 1851 to 1853. Mendel spent most of his time there learning physics, mathematics, and chemistry. He studied physics with Christian Doppler, well known for the Doppler principle, as well as with other distinguished experimental physicists. From them he learned the skills and methods that were to be so important in his later research. Above all, it was the fundamental philosophy of the physics department that complex phenomena could be reduced to laws of nature, often based on particles of matter. Designing experiments to discover and clarify these laws of nature was the principal feature of the department. Mathematics and statistics were obviously essential whenever the results were quantitative.

Upon his return to Brno, Mendel applied the principles of physics and mathematics to the investigation of heredity in plants. Looking back with the advantage of hindsight, we can see that his experimental designs and many of his conclusions were awe inspiring. It is also evident that he pioneered the use of statistics in biological research.

Mendel's research was a part-time affair, done in addition to his usual activities as a monk. Despite this limitation, with an experimental plot and a new greenhouse he grew twenty-eight thousand plants between 1854 and 1863. A crucial aspect of his work was that he always started by reducing each problem to its component features—comparable to the particles of matter in physics research. All the individual characteristics of the plants he studied were investigated separately.

In one well-known experiment he crossed plants with round seeds and plants with angular seeds. The result: the next generation had 5,474 round seeds and 1,850 angular seeds—a ratio of approximately 3 to 1. From this and other experiments Mendel concluded that reproduction was not a diffuse merging of characteristics from both parent plants, as was believed at the time. He decided instead that discrete particles conveyed the messages of heredity from one generation to the next. It was not until fifty years later that Mendel's particles were named "genes."

He also concluded that, in reproduction, a single cell from one parent fused with a single cell from the other parent. To explain the 3-to-1 ratio, he called the particles (or genes) from the round seeds "dominant" and those from the angular seeds "recessive." Thus, two parents with particles AA and aa would have offspring whose particles were mingled at random: AA, Aa, Aa, and aa. Consequently, the three offspring with a dominant A would have round seeds, while only the single offspring with two recessive particles aa would have angular seeds. In this simplest form of Mendelian heredity two genes, one from each parent, determined the plant's characteristics.

Mendel went on to investigate characteristics determined by two or more genes. He decided that the color of garden plants obeyed a more complicated law, "which possibly finds expression through the combination of several independent color characters."

He presented this research to the Natural Science Society in 1865 in two lectures, the texts of which were subsequently published. Mendel knew that what he had discovered was of fundamental importance; but even though he was quoted from time to time, scientists did not understand the significance of his research until several years after his death in 1884. This sad fact illustrates that in research it is necessary not only to perform investigations and to draw conclusions, but also to explain the findings to the world—as did Pasteur, Metchnikoff, and Ehrlich. The extraordinary monk Mendel was far too humble for that.

When the structure of the genetic material DNA (deoxyribonucleic acid) was finally established in 1953 by James Watson and Francis Crick, the publicity and the emotional reaction were so great that many people formed the impression that knowledge of nuclear material, the "secret of life," had begun at that time. That is far from true, but the story is an excellent example of how numerous investigators can make many discoveries over a long period before a particularly dramatic disclosure catches our imagination and leads to new worlds in science.

We *could* begin the DNA story in 1880, when it was generally agreed that, as a cell reproduces itself, division of the nucleus occurs before division of the rest of the cell. In the dividing nucleus were seen threads, first called "chromosomes" (meaning "colored bodies") in 1888. By then it was accepted that chromosomes are the bearers of heredity; we now know that each of us has twenty-three pairs of chromosomes and at least fifty thousand genes.

But we could just as well begin the DNA story back in 1869, when Fritz Miescher, a Swiss physiologist, isolated nucleic acid from nuclei. Following Miescher's lead, Albrecht Kossel isolated all the components of the nucleic acids (and in 1910 received a Nobel Prize for this work). About three decades later, using ultraviolet light to estimate the presence of DNA and RNA in cells, Torbjörn Caspersson and his associates in Stockholm showed that DNA is mainly in the chromosomes and connected with the reproduction of genes, whereas RNA is important in the synthesis of protein within a cell.

Then, in 1944, DNA researchers witnessed one of the supreme discoveries in the history of biology. Oswald T. Avery of the Rockefeller Institute in New York extracted nucleic acid (DNA) from one strain of bacteria and transferred it to another strain. By this means he showed not only that the second strain acquired the characteristics of the first, but that these characteristics were transmitted to subsequent generations, thus demonstrating the chemical and physical basis of heredity. Because of its far-reaching implications, this discovery earned for Avery the Copley Medal of the Royal Society in 1945. Moreover, his name was proposed for a Nobel Prize, which he did not receive because some experts doubted his conclusions. Years later, justice was done in a book (*Nobel: The Man and His Prizes*) edited by the Nobel Foundation, which noted: "Avery's discovery in 1944 of DNA as carrier of heredity represents one of the most important achievements in genetics, and it is to be regretted that he did not receive the Nobel Prize. By the time dissident voices were silenced, he had passed away."

Nucleotides have long been known to be essential constituents of chromosomes. Sir Alexander Todd (later Lord Todd) had been studying nucleotides for fifteen years when in 1957 he won the Nobel Prize for Chemistry for this research. Before his work in Cambridge the constituents of nucleotides were known, but not their means of combining. Using synthetic chemicals and intricate techniques, he constructed models of nucleotides that demonstrated how the sugars, bases, and phosphates are linked as a chain within nucleic acids. Erwin Chargaff, of the College of Physicians and Surgeons in New York, reported in 1950 that the paired constituents of DNA—adenine and thymine, and guanine and cytosine—were always equal in any species. His observations became known as "Chargaff's Rules," which were crucial in determining DNA's structure.

So many books, articles, and reviews have been written about the discovery of the structure of DNA that we can easily trace each step. This extensive, sometimes frank, literature also provides rare glimpses of the complicated social and psychological interactions among scientists. From that standpoint the most revealing accounts are *Rosalind Franklin and DNA* by Anne Sayre and *The Double Helix* by James Watson. A friend of Rosalind Franklin, Sayre describes with rare sensitivity a dedicated, shy, and attractive young woman encountering the loneliness and frustration that are all too frequent in a male-dominated institution. Maurice Wilkins had been studying DNA at King's College in London for a few years when Franklin arrived to work independently as an x-ray crystallographer and was advised to use her expertise to obtain patterns of crystals of DNA. Working almost in isolation, she produced several results that proved to be essential in determining the structure of DNA. It was her custom to work methodically, piling fact upon fact. When in 1953 she felt obliged to leave King's, she drafted an article based on her research. In that draft she deduced that in DNA the basic structure is a helix—very probably a double helix. She also concluded that the phosphate groups or phosphate atoms are on a helix with a diameter of about twenty angstroms, and that the sugar and base groups are on the inside of the helix.

In 1950 James Watson, a geneticist, and Francis Crick, a physicist, began to work together in the Cavendish Laboratory of Cambridge University, just as relevant information was becoming available from many quarters. Crick, being older and having a profound knowledge of physics, was the teacher; Watson was the pupil. As theorists, they did little laboratory research related to DNA; instead, they adopted an approach that was in many ways more difficult. They gathered all the evidence they could acquire by any means: from the literature, from meetings, from distinguished workers at the Cavendish, from many brilliant people in the extended Cambridge family, from an international network of experts in the field, from Maurice Wilkins, and (without her knowledge) from Rosalind Franklin. They then built everything that was known into one structure. This approach is a totally different process from the painstaking accumulation of scientific facts at the laboratory bench. Like all research workers, Watson and Crick made mistakes; but eventually, in 1953, they assembled a model of the structure of DNA that has withstood the test of time.

When they explained their conclusions to Wilkins and Franklin, it was agreed that Watson and Crick, Wilkins, and Franklin would submit three separate articles, which were published together in *Nature* on April 25, 1953. Franklin made only one addition to her earlier draft: "Our general ideas are not inconsistent with the model proposed by Watson and Crick." Years later Crick explained that when they submitted their first article, Watson had seen Franklin's x-ray evidence, but Crick had not. Yet Watson feared that their proposed structure was wrong and that he had made a fool of himself. Only after they read Franklin's article and appreciated how much she had done were they emboldened to write a second, more explicit article for *Nature*. In 1962, Crick, Watson, and Wilkins were awarded the Nobel Prize in Medicine and Physiology.

The tragedy is that Rosalind Franklin died of cancer in 1958, at the age of thirty-eight. Many wish that she had lived to be a candidate for the Nobel Prize. But, perhaps like others who deserve to win and do not, she would have been satisfied with her own knowledge of what she had achieved. Among the many lessons in this very human story is the necessity of working as part of a harmonious team in which ideas can be shared and developed by repeated discussion—a necessity that Watson and Crick enjoyed, but Franklin was denied. In retrospect, Crick has suggested that if Franklin had been able to continue at King's, she might have deduced the entire structure on her own within three weeks of the date of writing her draft.

Watson's candid book, *The Double Helix*, was not published until 1968, when he was forty. After colleagues criticized drafts that were obviously unfair to Rosalind Franklin (who by then had died), Watson added an epilogue in which he described his attitude toward a major problem in science that still persists today, although perhaps to a lesser degree: "We both came to appreciate greatly [Franklin's] personal honesty and generosity, realizing too late the struggles that the intelligent woman faces to be accepted by a scientific world which often regards women as mere diversions from serious thinking."

After this brief excursion through the history of genetics research, we come to four diseases that, although not necessarily caused by single genes, illustrate the type of genetics studied by Gregor Mendel: familial Mediterranean fever, cystic fibrosis, hemophilia, and gout.

Familial Mediterranean fever is an example of a human disease caused by a pair of recessive genes. This unpleasant condition, which includes arthritis, is largely but not entirely confined to peoples of Mediterranean stock. To understand it, one must know something of the history of the Jewish people. Contrary to common belief, Jews do not have a uniform ethnic background, but can be divided into the Ashkenazi and the non-Ashkenazi. The Ashkenazi come from central and eastern Europe. The non-Ashkenazi comprise the Sephardi and other groups, including

Iraquis and Yemenites. Familial Mediterranean fever is generally found in the Sephardi, who derive mostly from Jews who left Spain during the Inquisition. Many settled on the southern shores of the Mediterranean, and some eventually found their way to the Middle East; few emigrated to the United States.

Because most of the people affected by familial Mediterranean fever lived in isolated conditions, the disease did not emerge as an important entity until Israel was established as a nation and modern medicine became available there. Thus, in 1950 brief reports were assembled and many new cases were studied intensively in Israel. Since most patients were Jews, it was essential to ascertain their countries of origin. It turned out that many who had the disease were Sephardi whose families had emigrated from Morocco, Tunisia, Algeria, Libya, Iraq, Turkey, or Egypt.

The clinical appearance of familial Mediterranean fever is so characteristic that it is easy to recognize despite the absence of specific tests. Two-thirds of those with this painful condition begin to have symptoms during the first year of life; in most patients, the illness starts in childhood. The typical features are short, sharp, severe attacks of pain in the abdomen, joints, chest, or skin, usually accompanied by fever. Most individuals have all forms of the complaint at various times. Between attacks the people with this disease are usually perfectly normal. Suddenly they are smitten with an attack of agonizing pain, compelling them to take to their beds for a few days. Then they recover and return to their normal way of life—until the next attack.

In typical attacks of arthritis, usually only one joint is involved at a time, frequently a large one, such as the knee or ankle. There is fever, intense pain, gross swelling, and exquisite tenderness. On recovery, the joint returns to normal and x-rays show no changes—at least for the first several years of the disease.

In London we see a few people with this disease who have flown here for diagnosis. There are also rare examples of native British and American people who have the disorder. On one occasion I saw an Englishman who had a history of attacks of severe pain in the heel. When I asked how long he had had these attacks, he replied that he had started to have them as a baby. When I asked if anyone else in the family had the same symptoms, I was told that most members did. So it was that I came to examine a large family of English people living in rural Essex and suffering from familial Mediterranean fever. Despite such sporadic cases, virtually all our knowledge of this disease comes from Israel and the Middle East.

Cystic fibrosis is a devastating and comparatively common genetic disease, affecting quality of life and causing premature death. It, too, results from a recessive gene. In white populations one person in twenty has a single cystic fibrosis gene. Because the gene is recessive, that person does not develop the complaint but is simply a carrier of the gene. When two carriers marry, one in four of the children has two recessive genes and develops cystic fibrosis. The result: for white people the disease is present in 1 of 2,000 births. It is less common in Asians and in Africans.

Certain glands are affected in cystic fibrosis: especially those in the airways of the lungs, in the pancreas, and in the sweat glands of the skin. In the lungs, thick mucus forms in the airways, leading to repeated infection and gradual damage to the lungs. In the sweat glands, the salt content is high. Before 1939 the majority of children with cystic fibrosis died of infection before they were one year old. Now, owing to improved nutrition, antibiotics, physiotherapy, and heart and lung transplants, one-quarter of the people with this disease live more than thirty years.

It has been absorbing to follow the use of modern techniques in the search for the gene of cystic fibrosis. By 1985 the gene had been located on a particular part of the seventh chromosome. Four years later, by concentrating on that chromosome, investigators identified the gene, thus opening many opportunities for future research.

About twelve years ago I was approached by Margaret Hodson and Sir John Batten of the Brompton Hospital in London to help in the investigation of arthritis in young people with cystic fibrosis. Now that these patients were living longer, arthritis had become a troublesome feature. Before then there had been occasional reports of cases, but no systematic studies; so we decided to define the clinical issues. We found that of two hundred fifty patients with cystic fibrosis, thirty had arthritis. Ten had hypertrophic pulmonary osteoarthropathy, twelve had a unique episodic arthritis, and the remainder were difficult to classify with confidence.

Hypertrophic pulmonary osteoarthropathy is an interesting condition whose mechanisms we consider in a later chapter on the role of the nervous system in joint disease. It had been linked previously with either lung cancer or severe chest infection; therefore, it was regarded as a disorder of late adult life. Now it has an increasing association with cystic fibrosis in young people. In our group of patients this unusual type of arthritis was virtually confined to those with severe lung disease—and the average age at the onset of arthritis was twenty years.

Episodic arthritis is not associated with severe lung pathology and is present in young people whose lungs function well. The age of onset varies from five to twenty years. In many respects, attacks of episodic arthritis are remarkably like those in familial Mediterranean fever. Between attacks the joints are normal. Then, after a sudden onset, these young people are confined to bed, look utterly miserable, and are unable to move because of the severity of the pain. After an average of four days, they recover and their joints return to normal.

In speculating on the possible causes of this unique episodic arthritis, we know that it is not familial Mediterranean fever, even though there is a resemblance. We have suspected a form of reactive arthritis as a response to lung infection, but we had no evidence that this is correct. Also, we have considered the possibility of a second gene or a mutation that determines which people with cystic fibrosis develop arthritis. With the clinical features of the problem thus outlined, the time is ripe for detailed research.

Hemophilia is an uncommon hereditary disorder in which a specific defect results in poor blood clotting and excessive bleeding. It originates with a gene on a sex chromosome.

With rare exceptions, all normal women have two X chromosomes, whereas men have an X chromosome and a Y chromosome. Consequently, a single recessive hemophilia gene on a female X chromosome will cause no disease in the female because it is recessive. The female acts as a carrier. In the male, the hemophilia gene on the X chromosome causes disease because it is unopposed. So none of the women and half of the men in a family develop hemophilia. In a well-known example, Queen Victoria was a carrier and had eight children, of whom Leopold had hemophilia and Beatrice was a carrier. In the next generation, there were two carriers and two Lords with hemophilia. In the third generation, two more males were affected.

Arthritis in people with hemophilia results from repeated bleeding into the joint structures and into the synovial fluid. In a secondary manner the immune system responds, so changes seen under a microscope are similar to those found in any persistent arthritis such as rheumatoid arthritis. Blood in the synovial tissue and in the synovial fluid apparently is treated as if it were foreign. Thus, hemophilia is an example of a sex-linked mode of inheritance, and of an arthritis resulting from the host's own substances being essentially normal but in the wrong location.

In introducing *gout,* I am hard pressed to improve on the description by Thomas Sydenham (1624–1649), which was based on years of personal experience:

> The victim goes to bed and sleeps in good health. About two o'clock in the morning he is awakened by a severe pain in the big toe; more rarely in the heel, ankle, or instep. The pain is like that of a dislocation, and yet the parts feel as if cold water were poured over them . . . Now it is a violent stretching and tearing of the ligaments—now it is a gnawing pain, and now a pressure and tightening. So exquisite and lively meanwhile is the feeling of the part affected, that it cannot bear the weight of the bed-clothes nor the jar of a person walking in the room. The night is spent in torture.

The criticisms of this description that we would make today are that gout is often milder and less dramatic, especially in large joints, and that gout may affect the arms, especially the hands and wrists. Like familial Mediterranean fever and the acute episodes of cystic fibrosis, typical attacks of gout usually last only a few days and are followed by complete return to normal. The best reason for suspecting gout is a history of characteristic previous attacks.

The causes of gout are many and complicated. It is a metabolic disorder that results from too much uric acid (or urate). This excess may derive from overproduction in the body, lack of removal by the kidneys, or excess absorption from food in the intestines. The level of urate in the blood of an individual indicates whether that person may develop gout, but it is only a guide. Throughout any population one finds all grades of urate levels; only a small proportion of those with raised levels develop symptoms of gout. Consequently, when patients present to a physician with joint pains and raised levels of urate, less than half prove to have gout.

Gender and age are undoubtedly significant factors in causation. Gout is, or used to be, ten times as common in men as women. The onset is seldom before the age of thirty, after which the frequency increases with age.

The ancient Greeks were aware that heredity plays a part in gout. Raised levels of urate also run in families. Major difficulties arise, however, when we attempt to define the exact nature of the heredity. At one time it was thought that a single dominant gene controlled urate production, but that view is no longer accepted. We find rare examples of single genes being important in certain families, with different genes in different families; but this raises more questions because we cannot assume that these rare genes are relevant in the average case of gout. The present preference is for a hereditary component that results from a combination of genes—most of which have not yet been identified—as well as other host and environmental factors.

Ethnic differences relating to gout are obvious in populations of the Pacific Rim. Although increased frequencies of gout and of urate levels have been established for people living on the Pacific islands, a more striking difference is seen when islanders migrate to New Zealand, Hawaii, or the United States, where they are more likely to have gout and to become overweight. Perhaps they have an inborn defect that fails to handle the diet of their adopted country.

Kidney disorders may result in retention of urate. And blood and skin conditions with rapid turnover of cells and destruction of cell nuclei may also lead to excess urate. Food and alcoholic drink can induce gout and raise urate levels, but in both instances their influence is far less than the popular image would suggest. Being overweight is often associated with gout. Improvement in gout follows weight loss; but starvation and rapid weight loss make matters worse.

Drugs are particularly important. Even the humble aspirin causes retention of urate. The worst culprits are diuretics (used to rid the body of excess fluid in the treatment of high blood pressure or heart disease); today a quarter of all new cases of gout are caused by diuretics. This applies especially to older women, who seldom develop gout unless it is induced by medication. Far from typical, this version of gout in women may be insidious and chronic and often affects the hands.

In addition to long-term factors that increase urate, short-term factors can precipitate individual attacks. These include local injury, alcohol, drugs, diseases, and surgical operations.

Given that most people with raised levels of urate never have gout, what causes the attacks, and why was Thomas Sydenham tortured by pain in his feet at two in the morning? Regrettably, we still have no satisfactory response to these questions.

To explain the attacks, we know that the urate in the blood has no difficulty entering the joints, because it is soluble. In some people urate is deposited in the synovium as sodium salt (monosodium urate), and part of it enters the synovial fluid. During an attack of gout, crystals form in the synovial fluid by a chain reaction, as happens with any crystals in a fluid. The immune system sounds the alarm, and within a few minutes hordes of polymorphs are attracted to the scene to engulf the crystals. Many polymorphs are destroyed in the struggle and release their own powerful enzymes as well as the crystal debris, thereby intensifying the inflammatory response in the joint.

For Sydenham's symptoms of pain in the feet in the middle of the night there are many explanations, but one is more ingenious than the others. It is that the feet, being dependent throughout the day, swell with fluid that includes soluble urate. In the prone position in bed, the fluid is absorbed into the bloodstream more rapidly than the urate. The temporarily high concentration of urate is apt to result in precipitation and consequently in an attack of gout in the feet.

Compared with our complicated target diseases of ankylosing spondylitis, psoriatic arthritis, and rheumatoid arthritis, these four diseases, which can be partly or wholly explained by Mendel's laws, are relatively simple. The four diseases differ in other ways, including their frequent, sudden, brief attacks. It is apparent that if a hereditary element exists in our target diseases, it is not on the basis of "one gene, one disease." We need a more sophisticated explanation.

10

Joint Failure

When I first worked at the Royal National Orthopaedic Hospital in London, many conferences about patients were devoted to the difficult task of advising suitable surgical operations for joint failure due to severe disorders of the hip joint. Because of their disease, patients often were severely disabled and had to lead sadly restricted lives. Surgeons knew only too well that the operations they advised would be frequently unsuccessful; it was not unusual for brilliant surgery to result in continuing disability or pain and, all too often, further operations. Few patients were able to discard their walking sticks or canes and lead active lives again.

Times changed, and we entered a period that was in many ways more disappointing. The early attempts to make artificial hip joints, which held such promise, were ill conceived. Sometimes surgeons, lacking suitable advice, designed devices that paid insufficient attention to engineering principles. Artificial joints frequently failed within a few months of surgery and had to be replaced.

Two British orthopedic surgeons did more than anyone else to overcome these problems: Kenneth McKee in Norwich, and John (later Sir John) Charnley, who worked near Manchester. They collaborated with engineers and scientists to design joint replacements that were truly successful. For the first time, people crippled by hip disease could take to the dance floor within a few weeks of surgery.

This success was followed by a worldwide reorganization of orthopedic surgery. The result has been one of the most important therapeutic advances in the history of medicine. Literally millions of people have now had successful hip replacements. In North America alone, 120,000 hip-replacement operations are performed each year. Severe pain may be relieved immediately, and most patients go home after ten days. There follows a period of six to twelve weeks on crutches, and a further similar period of improvement before the patient feels fully fit and active.

Success with hip joints has been followed by success with knee joints, elbows, and shoulder joints. The period of development was longer for these joints because their structure and function are more complicated. Now knee replacements are virtually as satisfactory as the better-known hip replacements.

Joint failure is not a single disorder, but the final common pathway of a host of disorders. Put simply, in joint failure the cartilage and underlying bone become worn, a process that leads to local tissue reaction and nature's attempts at tissue repair. Expressed in those terms, the condition is easy to understand; unfortunately, it is made confusing and frightening by the title "osteoarthritis," a word I need to use and to explain. Like other unsatisfactory words, "osteoarthritis" means different things to different people.

You will remember that it was not until the beginning of the twentieth century that osteoarthritis was distinguished from rheumatoid arthritis. In large part, this distinction resulted from studying the pathology of the two conditions, especially under the microscope. "Osteo" was included in the word because of changes readily seen in bone, but, regrettably, "arthritis" was retained. Thus, the word implies that osteoarthritis is primarily a form of inflammation of a joint—which it is not. The unfortunate consequence is that today millions of people with worn joints believe that they have arthritis and are apt to become crippled. It is often difficult to alter that firmly held belief.

In osteoarthritis (the worn joint in Figure 13), the first changes include minute fissures on the surface of the joint cartilage. The diseased cartilage gradually becomes thinner, which leaves the ligaments long and sometimes makes the joint unstable. At the same time, the underlying bone is affected. It becomes denser, growing out at the sides in a primitive response to the damage. At first, evidence of inflammation in the synovium is minimal—only a small amount of extra synovial fluid;

later, minute fragments of cartilage and bone are shed into the synovial fluid and absorbed by the synovium. Because these fragments are diseased and in the wrong place, they induce a secondary inflammation in and around the synovium. As part of the response, the capsule and surrounding ligaments become loose or, alternatively, thickened and more rigid. In a stiff joint, these changes in the capsule and ligaments restrict mobility; surgical division of these structures around the joint often restores movement.

By contrast, in an inflamed joint (as with rheumatoid arthritis) the inflamed synovium becomes grossly thickened and the synovial fluid increases. The inflammation is not confined to the synovium but affects tissues around the joint, including the ligaments. Owing to the pressure within the joint and the physical strain of using the joint, the weakened supporting structures (including the ligaments) may stretch, and this development leads to excess movement or early deformity. Unlike osteoarthritis, rheumatoid arthritis is not primarily a disease of cartilage or bone, but at a later stage these structures may be invaded and damaged by inflammation. A characteristic feature of an inflamed joint is marked loss of substance in the neighboring bone.

Joint failure is not a passive process whose features simply result from use, age, and misfortune; it is highly dynamic—and, to researchers, definitely a challenge. Overcoming basic disease processes in joint failure

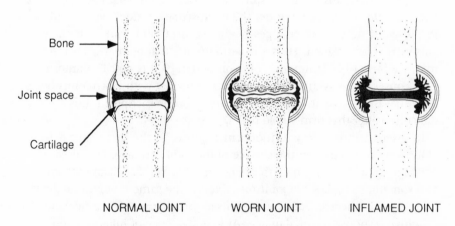

NORMAL JOINT   WORN JOINT   INFLAMED JOINT

Figure 13 • The essential features of normal, worn, and inflamed joints.

through new methods of prevention or treatment has become one of the most sought-after goals in medicine.

Joints fail for many reasons. As one would expect, the causes are cumulative in their effects, so osteoarthritis becomes more common with advancing years. By age fifty, half of the population exhibits signs of osteoarthritis on x-ray; and by age seventy, everyone has some abnormal joints.

There is a striking discrepancy between the anatomical changes in joints and the pain and disability they cause. For this reason, people should usually be guided by their symptoms and not be unduly worried by reports of the x-rays of their joints—provided that the joints are not troublesome. Fortunately, only about 20 percent of those with definite osteoarthritis have significant symptoms. The overall frequency of osteoarthritis varies with the definition used, but a reasonable estimate of those with troublesome symptoms caused by this type of joint disorder is 5 percent of the entire population—probably 12 million in the United States and 3 million in Britain.

When we consider the causes of osteoarthritis, we have the overwhelming impression that this is a subject waiting for a breakthrough, and that at any time new findings could reorient all our thinking. Let us start with something obvious: a joint may fail because of imperfect development, old injury, or previous disease. For example, when assessing patients with hip disease in later life, we may find a history of partial displacement of the joint at birth or in adolescence, or disease of the joint during childhood. Osteoarthritis may result from a previous fracture which, besides breaking the bone, has entered a joint and deformed it. Alternatively, there may have been temporary inflammatory arthritis in early adult life. And, of course, mild, persistent arthritis may have led to joint failure. Prevention of these types of joint failure is one of the prime purposes of all treatment of bone and joint disorders. Although this approach has been highly successful, it does not illuminate our search for fundamental causes.

The first clue to the presence of an inherent underlying disorder lies in the fact that joint failure, unless caused by a previous injury or disease, is usually symmetrical. For instance, a high proportion of people requiring hip-replacement surgery eventually have operations on both sides. So we are not considering a random process of wear and tear.

The next clue is that there are patterns to the kinds of joints affected. Furthermore, these patterns are not confined to individuals but are found widely in families and in certain races. Although some of these racial characteristics are undoubtedly due to postures adopted as a matter of custom (squatting, for instance), there is strong evidence of hereditary factors.

We have now raised, for the first time, the basic question of why certain joints are affected in particular disorders and in particular individuals. There must be answers, but as yet we do not know which of several explanations is correct. Because in osteoarthritis we have good reason to favor a dominant role for heredity, let me briefly review the genetic control in the embryo that makes our joints symmetrical to begin with.

At the end of the fourth week after successful fertilization of a human ovum, the arms and legs begin as buds on the sides of the embryo. Following genetic instructions, both arms grow from the trunk and eventually form adult arms and hands—perfect in size, shape, and structure, and each a precise mirror image of the other. The fingerprints are virtually identical, yet they are sufficiently specific to identify a single individual. Of special importance to us is the knowledge that the genetic information in the fertilized ovum determines the formation of each joint and ensures that it is a mirror image of its counterpart in the opposite limb.

Although we do not yet know all the details of the process, our genes direct embryonic cells to multiply in different parts of the body. Having reached their destinations, the cells are secured in place, directed to take on new forms, and ordered to build complicated structures such as bones, joints, and muscles. When each item is exactly correct, the cells are instructed to stop. This process continues for the rest of our lives; cells are constantly replaced and each tissue and organ must be maintained as originally directed in our genetic blueprints. The process is not perfect, however. After injury or removal of a part of the body, our genes supervise excellent repairs; but their capacity to do so is more limited than in less complicated creatures. So, if our genes can make our fingerprints exactly alike, it is not too much to imagine that they can also determine whether matched pairs of joints remain intact—or fail in unison.

In addition to symmetry and patterns of disease, some joints in the body regularly escape disease, whereas others are unusually vulnerable: osteoarthritis is common in the big toe, at the base of the thumb, at the ends of the fingers, in the knees, and in joints of the spine; it is rare in the wrists, elbows, shoulders, and ankles. The usual explanation is that susceptibility depends on the physical design of these joints. In some, there is "discongruity," which means that the joints do not fit accurately as a result of the way they were constructed in development. As with symmetry and joint patterns, some families and some races frequently differ from normal in the design of their joints and in their tendency to joint failure.

In 1802 an English physician, William Heberden the Elder, described small nodules near the end joints of the fingers. These are created by excess bone associated with osteoarthritis of the local joints. We now know that "Heberden's nodes" either follow minor injuries or are spontaneous. When spontaneous, they are more frequent after the age of forty-five years and almost exclusive to women. They usually cause few symptoms, but they may be uncomfortable in the early years and occasionally they are very painful.

Heberden's nodes tend to be part of a generalized process of osteoarthritis and hence are of considerable theoretical interest. A distinguished American rheumatologist, Robert Stecher, first established a strong hereditary component in spontaneous Heberden's nodes: in the families of people with this type of Heberden's nodes, many close relatives have the same condition. Later Jonas Kellgren in England showed that the distribution of joints affected by generalized osteoarthritis varies according to the presence of Heberden's nodes.

Kellgren and his colleagues also made two interesting observations about people with generalized osteoarthritis who did not have Heberden's nodes. Their study demonstrated no female preponderance and showed a definite increase in the frequency of rheumatoid arthritis in close relatives. These findings could be interpreted as meaning that genes for rheumatoid arthritis in a family can predispose to osteoarthritis, with a distribution of joint involvement in the hands similar to that of rheumatoid arthritis—an intriguing possibility.

Following the lead that osteoarthritis may have a hereditary component, several researchers have investigated families whose inheritance of osteoarthritis is strong. In these special families osteoarthritis is linked to a gene that controls a certain class of connective tissue (type 2 collagen). This gene is known to be on the twelfth chromosome. But because only rare, exceptional families were investigated, it would be wrong to assume that a gene has been discovered for the more common forms of osteoarthritis.

Next, we come to the role of female hormones. In women many joints may be affected by a generalized process of severe osteoarthritis. Two American physicians, Russell Cecil and Benjamin Archer, in 1925 described a form of chronic arthritis in overweight, middle-aged women. The disorder occurred at or just after menopause and was characterized by persistent pain and stiffness in the joints affected. Cecil and Archer gave it the unfortunate name "menopausal arthritis," a term that has survived within folklore but in such a confused way that its current usage no longer relates to the condition it originally described.

Several years later this disorder was reinvestigated and renamed "primary generalized osteoarthritis," because it was found to belong to a wider age group and was not especially associated with menopause. Its onset is rapid, with a mean age of fifty-two years. Twenty percent of those afflicted had the disease before menopause. Many joints were affected—particularly hands, knees, and spine. Again, obesity was a common feature. (We return to this disorder in the next chapter, when we consider whether hormones affect its progress.)

It is a common fallacy that worn joints should be exercised vigorously to prevent their becoming stiff. While it is true that judicious exercise, notably swimming, is helpful, millions of people who think physical activity will help them only succeed in making their joints far worse by doing too much. Many occupations and sports have led to undue wearing of joints. A Swiss group investigated long-distance runners, bobsled riders, and healthy, untrained men. They were examined and x-rayed in 1973 and again in 1988. Fifteen years after the initial assessment, the runners had significantly more osteoarthritis of the hips, and this correlated well with the speed and distance of their running in 1973.

Now let us examine, in a different way, the intriguing possibility that osteoarthritis may be part of a generalized disease. I start by recounting a research project that emphasized the biological activity of joint cartilage. The results dispelled the common misconception that cartilage and bone, which are the most important structures in osteoarthritis, behave as if they were dead and without function. These structures are alive and do not simply wear, as mechanical parts do.

Our story concerns an able young medical graduate, Ronald Jubb, and a doyenne of British medical science, Dame Honor Fell. Before he came to work in Cambridge in 1975, Jubb had graduated in Glasgow and completed his training in internal medicine. Dame Honor had retired five years before as director of the Strangeways Laboratory in Cambridge, but she was still working seven days a week.

In scientific discovery it is often a positive advantage to come fresh to a subject. Dame Honor was studying the effect of enzymes on the breakdown of joint tissues, and Jubb joined her project from a background in clinical internal medicine. Thus, his mind was not constrained by current views on the role of enzymes in joints; he felt, at that stage, that any cell could do anything. Dame Honor, released from administrative responsibilities, was free to pursue her pioneering work on organ culture. Not only did she have a reputation for obsessional, personal attention to detail in laboratory work, she had established a system for maintaining mature joint tissues in culture.

The two investigators formed an ideal team: the one young and unprejudiced, the other elderly and experienced. Not only did this combination bode well for the project's success, but Fell and Jubb elected to study a tissue with only one type of cell. Unlike other forms of cartilage in the body, adult joint cartilage contains only chondrocytes (cartilage cells). That decision was crucial to the interpretation of their results.

Jubb obtained fresh trotters, or pigs' feet, from the local slaughterhouse, where suitable pigs were often killed at 6:30 a.m. He then dissected some synovium and joint cartilage and set them up in organ culture. Isolated cartilage in culture normally remains alive and intact for several weeks, whereas in similar conditions synovium destroys itself and digests its connective tissue, leaving a mass of living cells.

When live synovium was placed on live cartilage, the cartilage beneath the synovium underwent an unexpected severe breakdown. At first, Honor and Jubb assumed that enzymes from the synovium were responsible, but then they noted that the breakdown was much more rapid and extensive if the chondrocytes were alive. Apparently the chondrocytes played an active role in the destruction.

When the experiment was repeated, this time separating the synovium and the cartilage so that synovial enzymes were inactivated by the intervening medium, the chondrocytes digested the cartilage matrix between the cells and destroyed a considerable portion of the cartilage. Much later, the chondrocytes changed their appearance to resemble other cells, and the whole picture was reminiscent of rheumatoid arthritis. The nature of this communicating factor—one that could turn chondrocytes into such destructive cells—was then investigated at Strangeways. Although called catabolin for a while, the factor discovered by Fell and Jubb proved to be the same as another factor, interleukin-1.

After this set of experiments, it was clear that joint cartilage could no longer be regarded as the passive victim of destruction. The seemingly lowly, inert chondrocytes could be transformed by humoral factors and play an active role in destroying the matrix of the cartilage.

This relatively simple biological research has had profound implications for our understanding of the function of normal and diseased joints. Since 1977, when the work was first published, worldwide research has been intense and has resulted in much helpful, though highly technical, information. By 1989 chemicals were developed to block the action of interleukin-1. This breakthrough provided the exciting prospect of drug therapy that can reduce joint destruction.

Three uncommon conditions illustrate the important principle that joint failure can result from generalized, apparently remediable disorders. The first condition, described in 1887 by Vicenzo Brigidi, was called acromegaly—meaning large limbs. At the postmortem of a patient, Brigidi noted a marked enlargement of the pituitary gland on the underside of the brain. (We now know that in this patient a slow-growing tumor of the pituitary gland would have produced an excess of growth hormone. Because the patient was an adult whose bones and joints were fully formed, the growth hormone would have caused the bone, cartilage, ligaments, and other structures to enlarge rather than to grow in length.) From our point of view, what is interesting about this condition is that the bone, cartilage, and ligaments, though larger, are of poor quality. Because the bone and cartilage are weak, they wear and give rise to osteoarthritis in some joints; and because the ligaments are weak, other joints are loose and unstable. This is an excellent example of multiple joint failure caused by excess of a natural hormone.

Three decades ago, while working in Philadelphia, Daniel McCarty investigated the synovial fluid of patients with gout. He discovered calcium pyrophosphate dihydrate in the synovial fluid of several patients whose gout was atypical. In doing so, he rediscovered a little-known disease and called it pseudogout. Later the same chemical was found to mimic chronic arthritis, such as rheumatoid arthritis. At other times it caused attacks so abrupt and severe that they resembled acute infection of the joints by live bacteria. In many individuals the process was much more insidious. Crystals of this chemical were deposited in the cartilage of the joints, which in turn weakened the cartilage and led to osteoarthritis. This situation typifies multiple joint failure caused by a metabolic process.

Between 1840 and 1860 a previously unknown condition was identified among Cossacks who lived in an eastern area of Russia, near Lake Baikal between the Argun and Shilka rivers. It was also present throughout eastern Siberia, northern China, and northern Korea. This disorder was first described in 1849 and now bears the name Kashin-Beck disease.

Children of school age were affected. They gradually developed severe, symmetrical damage to the cartilage and bone in many of their joints, followed by osteoarthritis, especially in the hands, elbows, knees, and feet. This terrible condition did not run in families; curiously, the local people noticed that it was more frequent after wet harvests. Furthermore, adults who moved into the area developed a modified form of the disease. It clearly had the hallmarks of a disease caused by something in the environment rather than by something inherited. The conclusion at the time was that the disease resulted from eating cereal grain infected with the fungus *Fusaria sporotrichiella*. The frequency of arthritis was reduced considerably by importing cereals from other countries, including Canada. Kashin-Beck disease fortunately is now much less common in Russia and is even said to have disappeared.

This ailment has been investigated more recently by the Chinese. For several decades they have suffered from a wide distribution of Kashin-Beck disease affecting between 1 million and 5 million individuals out of a local population of 30 million Chinese in a belt that includes the northeast, the northwest, Tibet, and Qinghai Province. This tragic swath of severe joint disease in children extends for more than twenty-five degrees of latitude. The children at risk are six to thirteen years of age, with up to 70 percent of children afflicted in some regions. Although those at risk live mostly in mountainous agricultural regions, the condition is also found in the Songnen and Songliao plains. The frequency of children with joint disease has varied from year to year, and from season to season. Also, the disease frequency sometimes diminishes in one endemic area at the same time that it rises in other endemic areas; but the movement of Kashin-Beck disease from endemic to nonendemic areas does not resemble the spread of an infectious disorder. Affected children who have left endemic areas are said to improve and develop normal x-rays after six to twelve months.

Maize and wheat, but not rice, are believed to be crucial factors in the distribution of the disease. In 1972, it was reported that cereals in the endemic areas were deficient in the nonmetallic element selenium. A few years later, public concern led to a formal epidemiological study authorized by the Ministry of Health. Selenium levels were found to be high in the southeast and northwest of China, and low in between. Kashin-Beck disease was distinctly more common in three hundred counties in fourteen provinces, with reports of good correlation between disease and selenium deficiency.

Where the content of selenium in drinking water is low, the selenium levels in individuals depend largely on their food. Meat, eggs, and rice raise selenium levels, as measured in the urine. Unfortunately, the food of children in endemic areas of China consists largely of corn, wheat, and highland barley—all deficient in selenium. The distribution of selenium-fortified salt to schoolchildren, begun in 1974, gave encouraging results. But the belief that selenium is the sole cause of the disease has been largely abandoned; disease has occurred where the availability of selenium is higher than usual, and *no* disease has been found in some areas where there is severe selenium deficiency.

Infection of wheat and maize by two different fusaria, *Fusaria oxysporum* and *Fusaria moniliforme,* has been investigated by the Kashin-Beck Institute in China. Researchers there suspect that other agents in the disease are toxic products of fusaria, including one called threitol, which is found only in endemic areas (but not in all of them). Another conclusion is that families in endemic areas who have poor sanitation and grow their own cereals as staple foods are especially at risk of developing Kashin-Beck disease. The primitive methods used for storing grain have attracted attention, with the thought that improved facilities might reduce the infection of maize and wheat. It is already known that importation of high-quality cereals is effective in the prevention and treatment of this common joint disease.

The appalling evidence from China, so carefully investigated, is a salutary reminder that other types of malnutrition may be extremely important, not only in deprived countries but in deprived groups of people anywhere. Of course, the story of Kashin-Beck disease, however intriguing, does not imply that selenium deficiency—or a vegetarian diet—

causes osteoarthritis in other areas. Indeed, there is evidence that the intake of selenium in people with arthritis elsewhere is normal. Nor is there reason to suspect that poor storage of grain causes joint disease in other parts of the world. Nevertheless, further research in China may prove to have immense implications for many common joint diseases.

— You will have noticed that, in both inflammatory arthritis and osteoarthritis, the frequency of different types of disease varies markedly with age and sex. Let us now review the possible explanations for this remarkable variation.

11

Age and Sex

Many disorders throughout medicine occur at a certain age or predominantly in one sex. We all rely heavily on this knowledge in making diagnoses; regrettably, we have become so accustomed to these facts of life that we sometimes cease to question why several million people suffer diseases of all kinds to which they would have been less susceptible if they had been a different age or sex. Although excellent research has been done on this topic, in general it has been sorely neglected.

In some types of arthritis, a man seventy years of age is a thousand times more susceptible than a woman of fifty, or a girl of three is a thousand times more susceptible than a man of forty. Here are two major clues that must be taken into account when reviewing the causes of arthritis.

If there is one aspect of arthritis that is distressing to everyone, it is the sight of a small child pitifully disabled by painful, swollen joints. It is a relief to know that rheumatic fever has almost disappeared from developed countries, and hence persistent arthritis in children is uncommon. But it certainly occurs: the frequency of persistent arthritis in Britain as recently as 1963 was estimated to be at least 600 per million children under the age of fifteen years, and possibly three times that figure.

"Systemic arthritis" constitutes a quarter of childhood cases. The average age of onset is five years, but onset even in adult life is something all rheumatologists have met. Many joints are affected and patients endure a generalized illness with fever, rash, and other characteristic features. Often it is a sad condition to treat.

In another quarter of children with arthritis, also with an average age of onset of about five years, either one joint is affected or a few joints, and the generalized features of systemic arthritis are absent. The majority of these children do well, but some have an insidious onset of eye inflammation, necessitating careful surveillance.

The third quarter of the children have a mixture of types of arthritis, including the arthritis associated with psoriasis or chronic bowel disease.

True rheumatoid arthritis (with all the characteristics of adult rheumatoid arthritis, including rheumatoid factor) occurs in 10 percent of children with persistent arthritis. The average age of onset in this group is eleven years, and girls are affected twice as often as boys. Of these children, most do well and have little residual disability provided expert treatment is available. But in some children the disease is progressive and far more troublesome.

That leaves just over 10 percent with ankylosing spondylitis. A typical onset, which I saw often at the Royal National Orthopaedic Hospital, is in a boy of about ten. Almost invariably, only one or two joints in the feet or legs are involved, with typical swelling and pain due to arthritis; but the spine is entirely normal—despite the diagnosis of ankylosing spondylitis. If these youngsters are followed into adult life, many develop spinal symptoms at the age of eighteen or soon thereafter. One of the unsolved mysteries of rheumatology is why a single disease behaves so differently depending on the age of the person.

The age of onset of acute anterior uveitis (with or without arthritis) is similar to ankylosing spondylitis, being rare before eighteen and commonly having an onset between eighteen and twenty-five years. In ankylosing spondylitis, and even more clearly in acute anterior uveitis, it is as if some enabling factor were switched on shortly after the age of eighteen is attained.

As we leave childhood, the pattern of disease frequency gradually alters with the years, like a kaleidoscope turning very slowly. In adolescence, either psoriasis or its arthritis may precede the other, so it may be several years before the two can be put together to make the diagnosis of psoriatic arthritis. Compared with rheumatoid arthritis, this type of arthritis is more evenly spread over the decades; thus physicians are especially mindful of psoriatic arthritis when examining young adults.

In ankylosing spondylitis, reactive arthritis, and acute anterior uveitis many of the most troublesome symptoms occur between the ages of eighteen and thirty-five. Hence, when a young adult of either sex pre-sents with, say, a painful swollen knee, doctors always consider this group of diseases.

Rheumatoid arthritis can begin at any age between five and ninety-five, but the most frequent onset is between thirty and sixty years, in both women and men. During middle age it is undoubtedly the domi-nant type of arthritis encountered by clinicians.

Arthritis frequently affects elderly people, but for several reasons the consequences are not the same as if they were younger.

Contrary to popular belief, it is possible for rheumatoid arthritis to begin after age seventy or eighty. The onset in such patients may be ex-plosive, with more systemic upset, more muscle pain, and more disabil-ity than is usual in young adults. Therapy with modest doses of cortisone-like drugs may be lifesaving; people confined to bed often re-cover quickly, thereby enabling the physician to reduce and then with-draw the treatment after a few weeks or months. Polymyalgia rheuma-tica is almost exclusively a disease of older people, as we have already seen. Several diseases, such as gout and osteoarthritis, are cumulative in their effects and become more frequent with increasing age. And indi-vidual patients who are very old may have a confusing mixture of dis-eases and disabilities.

Social circumstances and attitudes toward disease are sometimes im-portant factors in determining whether retired individuals seek medical advice about their symptoms. Some old people believe that rheumatic pains are an inevitable part of aging, and they are remarkably long-suffering and uncomplaining about severe, disabling conditions. At the other extreme, a few elderly folk, perhaps overcome by the many gen-eral problems of old age, present with minor physical conditions of little consequence, in reality seeking help with their social and emotional problems rather than their aches and pains.

Most old patients who have definite arthritis are exceptionally coop-erative and understanding. But because scientific knowledge of arthritis is recent, some patients have fixed ideas about causes and treatment. They often cannot be shaken from the mistaken opinion that their prob-lems are caused by acid, or dampness, or food; nor can they be dis-suaded from aggravating their pain by taking too much exercise, to "work it off." Strange and expensive remedies are sometimes preferred to orthodox treatment. And, in some old people, loneliness, depression, bereavement, frustration, and fear of death conspire to make pain less bearable and support more necessary.

*   *   *

Several proposals have been made to account for the influence of age (see Figure 14), but none has been substantiated. The most attractive suggestion is that sophisticated elements of the immune system mature and are more (or less) effective at different stages of life, just as plants flower in different seasons. When one considers the alternative notion that disease is caused by differing environmental and social circumstances at various ages, it is necessary to think of the widely varying customs and circumstances throughout the world. There is very little evidence that these circumstances alter the average age of onset in different communities (as it does in poliomyelitis, for example).

Nevertheless, viral and other infections do occur at different ages. First come infections within the uterus and in the newborn period. Next are infectious diseases in childhood, such as measles and mumps, which have been suggested as possible causes of certain unexplained diseases of adult life. Supporting evidence is incomplete, however, and this mechanism probably does not apply to most forms of arthritis. School attendance brings exposure to a new range of infections. Later, kissing

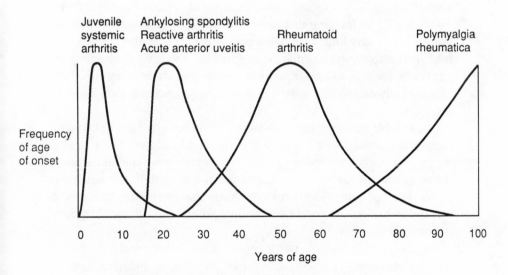

Figure 14 • This schematic graph illustrates the main differences in the age of onset in juvenile systemic arthritis, ankylosing spondylitis, reactive arthritis, acute anterior uveitis, rheumatoid arthritis, and polymyalgia rheumatica.

in adolescence transmits other viruses, such as the Epstein-Barr, which causes glandular fever. A little later, greater sexual activity leads to the spread of the common herpes viruses that infect almost all adults and remain concealed in the body for the remainder of life, except when they produce symptoms (as with mouth or genital herpes). There is little evidence that such viruses are primary agents in the causation of arthritis, but it is at least conceivable that in some diseases they might influence the age of onset during early adult life.

However hard I try, I cannot persuade myself that environmental factors play more than a secondary role in determining the overall pattern of different types of arthritis as they occur at certain ages in populations everywhere in the world. I prefer the suggestion that the changing susceptibility throughout life is caused by shifting populations of lymphocytes (or other cells), which increase, decrease, or become more or less effective according to the age of the individual. This hypothesis raises the intriguing possibility that the joints affected at different ages may be a function of individual joints having different, but changing, populations of cells.

The wide range of sex ratios in the frequency of various types of arthritis makes it easy to imagine that several factors may be involved. Indeed, there are so many biological differences between men and women that it is unwise to jump to simplistic conclusions about why this complex pattern exists. It is also necessary to consider the whole spectrum of sex ratios, as illustrated in Figure 15, rather than concentrate on a single disease at a time.

One reliable study suggests that women who have had few or no pregnancies are more likely to develop rheumatoid arthritis. Yet a similar report that the contraceptive pill may play a preventive role in reducing the frequency of rheumatoid arthritis has not been fully substantiated. Better, but not conclusive, evidence shows that hormone replacement therapy improves the course of rheumatoid arthritis, although it does not prevent its onset.

Pregnancy undoubtedly has a profound influence on the course of rheumatoid arthritis. After about two months of pregnancy, most women with this disease improve markedly, even though they have stopped all of their medication. The improvement is maintained until two or three months after delivery. By contrast, women with psoriatic arthritis or ankylosing spondylitis do not experience a similar improvement during pregnancy. The reason for this striking temporary improvement in rheumatoid arthritis is still unclear, although there has been a recent suggestion (to which we will return in a later chapter). As we have seen, systemic lupus erythematosus (SLE) occurs almost exclusively in women during childbearing years. There is also a tendency for SLE to start, or to worsen, during or soon after pregnancy.

I might note here that uterine fibroids and abnormal uterine bleeding are known to be associated with high levels of estrogen. A careful follow-up study of women with these conditions who had had a hysterectomy revealed that they were twice as likely to develop generalized osteoarthritis. This evidence, coupled with the fact that the condition affects mainly overweight, middle-aged women, strongly suggests that hormones play a part.

Excellent work has been done in experimental animals concerning the influence of female sex hormones on autoimmune disease. The findings suggest that sex hormones have a dominant role in the frequency of SLE, and probably in the severity of rheumatoid arthritis and some related diseases.

Next to consider is the influence of male-female differences in pelvic anatomy. As an example, men with gonorrhea develop a urethral discharge that is usually diagnosed quickly and treated effectively. Women

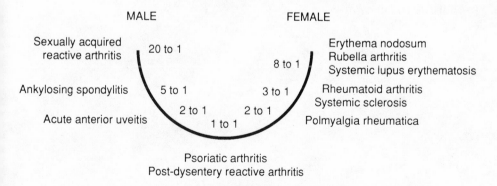

SEX RATIOS

MALE | FEMALE

Sexually acquired reactive arthritis — 20 to 1

8 to 1 — Erythema nodosum / Rubella arthritis / Systemic lupus erythematosis

Ankylosing spondylitis — 5 to 1

3 to 1 — Rheumatoid arthritis / Systemic sclerosis

2 to 1

Acute anterior uveitis — 2 to 1

2 to 1 — Polmyalgia rheumatica

1 to 1

Psoriatic arthritis
Post-dysentery reactive arthritis

Figure 15 • The range of sex ratios in the frequency of different types of arthritis.

with the same infection often have no pelvic symptoms and thus miss the opportunity for early diagnosis. Sometimes associated with menstruation or early pregnancy, the undetected infection in women can lead to gonococcal septicemia, which also is difficult to diagnose. The result may be infected blisters in the skin and arthritis of one or more joints owing to invasion by live bacteria. In this instance, the predominance of arthritis in women obviously depends on their pelvic anatomy.

The role of anatomy in reactive arthritis is more problematic. A man and a woman may have sexual intercourse and share the same microorganisms. After that, for reasons unknown, the man is twenty times as likely to suffer arthritis three weeks later. The same man and woman may eat eggs infected with salmonella and develop dysentery. In this situation they are equally likely to suffer arthritis three weeks later.

Even when we have allocated roles to sex hormones, pregnancy, and anatomy, we leave unanswered many questions relating to the spectrum of sex ratios, especially in diseases that occur predominantly in men. Why, for instance, is a ten-year-old boy five times as likely to have ankylosing spondylitis as a girl of the same age? This question raises the issue of genetics and whether sex chromosomes are responsible for modulating the entire spectrum of disease susceptibility—to the extent that tens of millions of people are more susceptible to arthritis than if they had been of the opposite sex. We have some but not all of the answers. The sex chromosomes contain many genes—far more than are required to determine gender. What these genes do, or may do, will be discussed later.

12

Other Common Causes of Pain

When anyone creates a service for the diagnosis and treatment of arthritis, he or she soon learns that it is not the doctors, or the managers, or those financing the service, who determine the type of patients to be treated. Unless there is some form of discrimination, it is the people with the diseases who apply for diagnosis and treatment and thereby define the service to be provided. It is also the people with the diseases who define the medical specialty of rheumatology. In keeping with that spirit, I write in this chapter about common nonarthritic conditions that are often described as "rheumatic" but are not part of any orderly scheme of diagnosis of arthritis. I start with the immense subject of backache and then describe a small selection of the innumerable other painful disorders that are frequently seen by rheumatologists—and by virtually all other doctors.

Spinal pain causing backache and neckache is a massive health-care problem. A recent population study in Britain showed that in one year 140,000 people per million consulted their general practitioners about spinal pain; and about 25,000 per million were referred to specialists. The implications of these figures deserve careful thought!

Conditions such as tumors and infections seldom manifest themselves as unexplained spinal pain, because the diagnosis is usually obvious from other symptoms. Similarly, it is unusual for arthritis (apart from ankylosine spondylitis) to present with symptoms in the spine. Minor congenital or developmental anomalies may explain the onset of pain in adolescence and in early adult life. Taken together, all of these diagnoses represent less than 1 percent of people with spinal pain.

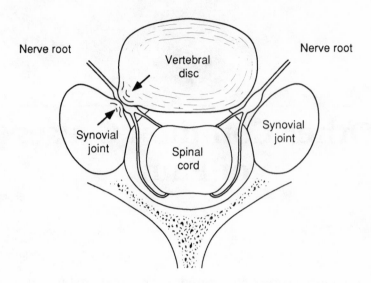

Figure 16 • An imaginary section through a vertebra in the neck, viewed from above.

More diagnostic problems are encountered with pain referred from the abdomen or chest. For example, gall bladder disorders may present with the gradual onset of discomfort between the shoulder blades, perhaps associated with indigestion. Kidney conditions may cause mild or severe pain in the lumbar region or a little higher; stomach ulcers may masquerade as lumbar backache; and so on.

After excluding serious disease, most doctors spend their time attempting to analyze the common causes of spinal pain. These causes can be divided broadly into those with symptoms due to pressure on nerve roots and those without such symptoms. Figure 16 shows a vertebra in the neck, as viewed from above. The spinal cord, within the spinal canal, is in the center. In front (the top part of the diagram) is the body of the vertebra, covered with a disc of cartilage. On either side are synovial joints; and at the back is the spine of the vertebra. The nerve roots emerge from the front and the back of the spinal cord. After traveling horizontally, they find their way out of the spine by passing through narrow canals on each side of the body of the vertebra and its disc. In the neck it is in these canals that the nerves are vulnerable to pressure from a disc or synovial joint, or both. If fluid forms in the synovial joint (as in a swollen knee), or a small protrusion of the disc develops, the nerve root may be compressed.

For comparison, Figure 17 illustrates the lower lumbar spine as seen from the side. At the lumbar level of the spine, the spinal cord has divided into many nerves, called the cauda equina (because it is similar to a horse's tail). In the figure, a nerve root (at the top) penetrates the thick lining that surrounds the cauda equina and travels down through the height of a vertebra before emerging from the spine. During that descent it is held tightly between the thick lining of the cauda equina and the lining of the vertebrae and the intervening disc. Hence, it is held taut exactly where it is apt to be compressed by a bulging disc.

A common misconception is that a disc "slips," like a washer emerging from between two bones the size and shape of cotton reels. What happens is nothing like that—anywhere in the spine. From adolescence on, discs become less liquid and less elastic, and their tough outer fibers tend to wear and give way. If a disc becomes worn and bulges, it is rather like a minute hernia, so there is no question of clicking it back into place. Instead, Nature gradually reduces the local swelling and replaces it with

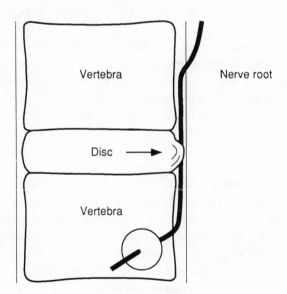

Figure 17 • Two vertebrae of the lumbar spine, seen from the side. At the top of the diagram, a nerve root penetrates the thick lining; it emerges one vertebra lower.

scar tissue that slowly shrinks. This is why recovery from nerve root compression takes weeks, or even months.

There is another difference between nerve compression in the neck and in the lumbar spine. In the neck, the little canal containing the nerve root enlarges when the neck is bent forward or rotated to the side, so root pain is usually relieved in that position. By contrast, a lumbar root joins the sciatic nerve and passes down the back of the leg into the sole of the foot. This anatomical arrangement gives rise to the diagnostic test in which the knee on the painful side is kept straight while the whole leg is moved forward. With lumbar root compression, this maneuver causes pain by stretching the nerve root over the protruded disc.

When a nerve root is compressed at any level of the spine, diagnosis is easier: pressure on each root leads to a characteristic distribution of symptoms in one arm, in the trunk, or in one leg. On examination, there may be areas of numbness, or local weakness of muscles, or changes in local reflexes. Any of these findings makes it possible to localize the abnormality in the spine and to judge its likely cause. The terms "brachial neuralgia" and "sciatica" are often applied to pain in the arm or leg resulting from root compression.

Diagnosis is inevitably limited and much more difficult when persistent spinal pain occurs in the absence of serious disease, abnormal x-rays, or root compression; that is, troublesome local pain in the neck or lumbar region may be the only guide. The difficulty in defining the problem accurately is that the interface between one vertebra and another is a complicated, coordinated system comprising a disc, two synovial joints, and many ligaments, to say nothing of the nerves and muscles that control them. It is impossible for one part of the system to be abnormal without affecting the other parts. In these circumstances—persistent local pain without root compression—it is usually comparatively simple to apply clinical criteria to localize the cause of the pain to one or two neighboring vertebrae, but it is difficult to be more precise. Standard x-rays are important in excluding serious disease and structural changes, but unfortunately are of little value in localization. In fact, the part that shows an abnormality on x-ray is statistically less likely to be the site of the pain, and more likely to represent an old problem that has undergone a slow process of repair.

No one can determine the exact cause of pain in an individual patient: a few fibers may have torn in one of the ligaments (like a sprained ankle in miniature), or there may be a minor derangement in a disc or synovial joint. The most expert and experienced physicians and surgeons do not claim to make a correct diagnosis in more than 25 percent of such patients. Fortunately, noninvasive imaging techniques, such as computer tomography and magnetic resonance, today are transforming our ability to assess the causes of spinal pain in people requiring surgery.

Pain in the shoulder has three common causes: capsulitis around the shoulder joint, damage to the rotator cuff, or compression of a nerve root in the neck. "Capsulitis" is a strange condition in which there seems to be mild inflammation around, but outside, the main shoulder joint. It is not a form of arthritis, and it does not spread to other joints. The onset is often between the ages of forty-five and sixty-five years. The patient slowly becomes aware that the shoulder is uncomfortable and hurts at the extremes of range: perhaps she cannot put her hand above her head or behind her back. The doctor's usual finding is that the shoulder's movements are evenly restricted in all directions. After three or four months or a little longer, the pain subsides and the patient stops worrying about the restricted movement. After a year or more, the shoulder regains its normal movements.

Rotator cuff disorders derive primarily from the unusual design of the shoulder joint. Unlike the hip, which is a ball-and-socket joint with considerable stability, the shoulder is a loose joint principally held together by tendons. The tendons of several muscles interdigitate to form a cuff over the front, top, and back of the shoulder. These tendons control most movements of the joint and hold it together. The cuff often begins to wear at an early age, interfering considerably with work and athletic activities. The symptoms are usually brief, but they may continue and force the patient to adjust to a persistent minor disability. Sometimes a worn rotator cuff is the site of heavy calcification. Under ordinary circumstances this calcification causes no symptoms. But if calcified material escapes into the surrounding tissues, the pain may be agonizing and require immediate treatment. Having experienced this condition myself, in both shoulders, my preference is for surgical removal of the calcified material—as soon as possible!

The condition "tennis elbow," which seldom arises from playing tennis, is not as simple as is commonly thought. It is a painful, tender condition over the prominent bone just above the outer aspect of the elbow, with several distinct causes: local inflammation at the point where the main forearm muscle joins the humerus; pain referred from minor osteoarthritis within the elbow joint; compression of a nerve root in the neck causing localized pain at the elbow; or, less commonly, a minor nerve trapped near the elbow.

"Carpal tunnel syndrome," unrecognized until 1950, is now widely known. It results from pressure under a ligament (of little practical value) that connects two bones at the front of the wrist. The median nerve, and all the tendons that bend the fingers and thumb, pass under this ligament in a confined space between the ligament and the underlying bones. Some people have a smaller space than is customary, so that the median nerve is more easily compressed. Also, loose tissue around the tendons may swell at night—particularly after prolonged overuse or during pregnancy. A typical patient with this condition has no symptoms during the day or on first going to bed. An hour or two later, he or she wakes with painful tingling in the hand, usually—but not always— on the thumb side. It is often necessary to get up, move around, and shake the hand before it becomes comfortable again. Such episodes can strike several times during the night and are especially troublesome on first waking in the morning, when the fingers feel swollen.

The prognosis depends on whether the cause is temporary, such as overuse, tenosynovitis (inflammation around a tendon), or pregnancy, because symptoms fade as the cause disappears. When there is clinical evidence of local inflammation or swelling, a steroid injection (well away from the median nerve) usually brings lasting relief. But the condition should not be allowed to grumble on for months or years. Simple surgery gives excellent results: it requires only a small incision and division of the ligament. Although the carpal tunnel syndrome never leads to arthritis, it is a common complication of early rheumatoid arthritis: rheumatoid tenosynovitis may compress the median nerve and causes persistent searing pain and marked stiffness of the whole hand. I mention this because a single injection can completely relieve local symptoms.

"Trigger finger" is an apt name. The two tendons that bend an individual finger pass under retaining ligaments shaped like croquet hoops, so if local swelling occurs in one of the tendons, it becomes difficult for the tendons to move through the hoops. Because the muscles that bend the fingers have great mechanical advantage compared with the muscles that straighten the fingers, the swollen tendon passes one way but cannot return. The result is that either it gets completely stuck in a flexed position for several minutes or it returns with a sudden snap—hence the name. Tendon swelling is sometimes so marked that the finger is almost rigid and cannot be bent at all. In most patients the symptoms can be abolished by a local injection. Or surgical division of the retaining ligament gives excellent permanent relief.

Years ago my colleague Peter Blower examined fifty people who had presented with one or more trigger fingers at least ten years before. None of them had developed evidence of arthritis, indicating that trigger finger is definitely not a first sign of impending joint disease. Yet when I examined the hands of three hundred people with rheumatoid arthritis, 34 percent of them had experienced trigger fingers at some point after the onset of their arthritis, as part of the rheumatoid process.

Hip pain causes confusion, whether it results from common osteoarthritis of the hip or other causes. Surprisingly many people do not know where their hips are; for example, some women imagine that their hip joints are close to the point on the pelvis where they take measurements for their clothes. The normal site of pain arising in one hip is in the groin (which is near the hip joint) and down the front of the thigh, although it may be partly in the buttock. By contrast, unilateral pain arising in the lumbar spine is often felt over the buttock and the side of the pelvis, but not in the groin. Another difficulty in diagnosis is that hip pain is often felt in the knee, and not in the groin at all. Thus, it is important for a doctor to examine the hip in each patient with pain in the knee.

A condition of elderly people called trochanteric bursitis deserves special mention. Among those diagnosed clinically as having prolonged, severe hip disease requiring surgery, a few can move their hip joints freely but have marked pain and tenderness over the prominent bone at the side of the thigh and cannot sleep on that side. On examination there is local tenderness due to local, chronic inflammation. Once diagnosed, trochanteric bursitis is a pleasure to treat because most patients recover fully after one or two injections.

Sudden pain and swelling in a knee commonly occur in young adults as a consequence of mechanical derangements within the joint. In men, a torn cartilage (meniscus) or internal ligament is a frequent injury in contact sports; while in women, spontaneous lateral dislocation of the kneecap may result from a minor variation in the anatomical development of the knee. The whole problem of internal derangements of the knee has been transformed by the availability of modern arthroscopes. It is now simple to look about inside to discover exactly what is wrong.

Whereas previously it was necessary to remove a whole cartilage because it was not visible in its entirety during an open operation, today the surgeon can see far more and perform precise operations through the arthroscope. Like hip replacement, arthroscopy is one of the most important advances in joint surgery.

Two disorders of bone create major problems: osteoporosis and osteomalacia.

In childhood, bones grow rapidly in length and size. Then, during adolescence, the bones not only continue to grow but also acquire extra bone substance as they gain in density and strength. This accumulation of bone substance in adolescence varies among races and therefore may be influenced by heredity. Bone substance is gradually lost throughout adult life: inevitably, bones are thinner and weaker in old age, when their ultimate strength depends mainly on the individual's capacity to accumulate bone in adolescence and then to retain it throughout adult life. The loss of bone in adult life is faster in some people than in others; women lose more than men, and their loss accelerates at the time of menopause. This early gain and subsequent loss of bone during a lifetime is largely predetermined and is difficult to alter by treatment. Hormone replacement can slow, and even reverse, bone loss. There is no evidence, however, that calcium supplements prevent bone loss in people whose diet is already adequate.

In addition to the bone loss in otherwise fit people, enforced immobility, malnutrition, injury, or disease may be contributing causes. As an example, children and young adults confined to bed for months or years because of illness in past years suffered bone loss so severe that they developed bone deformities; the bone substance was never restored in later life. Our special interests, arthritis and its accompanying pain and disability, always result in some secondary bone loss.

Significant lack of bone substance is called osteoporosis, which implies that the chemical composition of the bones is normal but there is insufficient bone. A good guide to the progress of osteoporosis is loss of height due to shortening of the spine as a result of partial bone collapse.

Osteoporotic bones are weak and prone to fracture. Symptoms are largely confined to the spine. Collapse of a vertebra, usually above the waist, may cause sudden, intense pain in an older person. The more severe pain settles spontaneously after about six weeks; symptoms are then much milder until further collapse occurs, perhaps years later.

"Osteomalacia" means softening of the bones. Usually caused by a lack of vitamin D, it is the adult equivalent of rickets in infancy. Apart from malnutrition and racial predisposition, osteomalacia can occur with some diseases of the intestines and after stomach surgery. A mixture of factors, including diet and lack of sunlight, contribute to the high frequency of osteomalacia in elderly people, even in developed countries.

Osteomalacia is usually unsuspected and undiagnosed. Unlike the sudden spinal pain of osteoporosis, the symptoms of osteomalacia are widespread vague aches, mainly in the limbs. The bone pains in the arms and legs can be similar to those of arthritis, which is why rheumatologists see so many people with this disorder. Once diagnosed and treated, patients improve within hours.

Osteoporosis and osteomalacia are strongly associated with the hip fractures that have become so common in the older female population. Sometimes an elderly woman trips and breaks a weak bone; sometimes the weak bone breaks spontaneously and causes her to fall.

Taken together, the nonarthritic conditions reviewed in this chapter represent pain and disability in immense numbers of people. Although the causes of these disorders are not the same as those leading to arthritis, they too are subject to extensive research, much of which is highly encouraging.

We have reached another turning point. We have reviewed many diseases and potential environmental causes of arthritis, as well as various functions of the body that may influence whether an individual is susceptible to inflammation in the joints. In the next three chapters I explore other factors that are interrelated and potentially crucial, especially in determining when an individual is most susceptible to joint disease. These other elements include adrenal hormones (as an introduction to the neuroendocrine system), nerves and the nervous system, and psychological and social factors.

13

Adrenal Hormones

The adrenals, two small glands situated just above the kidneys, appeared in sixteenth-century anatomy drawings but no one knew what they did. When at the beginning of the eighteenth century the Academie des Sciences of Bordeaux offered a prize for an essay to be entitled "Quel est l'usage des glandes surrenals?" no prize could be awarded because no essays were submitted.

Although Richard Bright, a famous physician at Guy's Hospital in London, had reported a tuberculous adrenal gland as early as 1831, it was not until 1855 that Bright's colleague Thomas Addison wrote a monograph on eleven cases of adrenal disease. All the patients had had similar symptoms, all had died, and all were found—at postmortem—to have severe disease of both adrenal glands. In effect, Addison showed that we cannot live without adrenal glands. In his monograph (*On the Constitutional and Local Effects of Disease of the Suprarenal Capsules*), which caused him to be known as the father of endocrinology, Addison wrote:

> It will hardly be disputed that at the present moment the functions of the supra-renal capsules [adrenals], and the influence they exercise in the general economy, are almost or altogether unknown. The large supply of blood, which they receive from three separate sources; their numerous nerves, derived from the semilunar ganglia and solar plexus; their early development in the foetus; their unimpaired integrity to the latest period of life; and their peculiar gland-like structure—all point to the performance of some important office: nevertheless, beyond an ill-

defined impression . . . I am not aware that any modern authority has ventured to assign to them any special function or influence whatever.

At the time, Addison's views on an association between the adrenal glands and disease were opposed by most of the medical world. His reports were rejected, even by the Royal Medical and Chirurgical Society while he was its president. Worse still, some critics attributed the mortality rate in his syndrome to the quality of his medical care. Then the adrenal glands were neglected for forty years—until the first adrenal hormone, adrenalin, was isolated from the adrenal medulla.

Today we know far more, but not enough. The most important fact we have learned is that the adrenal glands are components of an elaborate system, dominated by the brain and by the hypothalamus and the pituitary gland at the base of the brain. Each adrenal gland consists of an inner and an outer part, both of which produce hormones. The inner part (medulla) is virtually an extension of the nervous system and secretes adrenaline (epinephrine). The outer part (cortex) is stimulated by hormones from the pituitary and secretes mainly cortisol (equivalent to cortisone). Although hormones were originally defined as chemical substances made by the endocrine glands and secreted into the bloodstream (to act as messengers in regulating the functions of distant organs), it is currently accepted that the term includes similar hormones that convey messages to neighboring cells, or even to the cell that made them.

The hypothalamus, located at the base of the brain, has many intricate nerve connections with the brain. Moreover, the hypothalamus is connected with the peripheral nervous system, including the adrenal medulla, and also with the pituitary gland, to which it transmits releasing factors (hormones) by way of a special blood supply. The pituitary responds by dispatching any of several hormones destined for distant organs, including the adrenal cortex. In response, the adrenal cortex secretes hormones that damp down the activity of the pituitary gland by a servo or feedback system. It is an elaborate and finely balanced system.

A central figure in this work was an American physiologist, Walter B. Cannon. Born at Prairie du Chien on the upper Mississippi River in 1871, Cannon received his medical degree from Harvard in 1900 and six years later became Professor of Physiology at Harvard Medical School. Cannon's first major interest was in movements of the stomach and intestines. He studied their nervous control and the effects on them of emotional states. Next, he turned to the many functions of the adrenal glands. Here his primary interest was in how our organs, tissues, cells, and chemicals maintain equilibrium and restore the normal balance after unusual activity.

In one of his experiments he denervated an animal's heart so that it could not respond to nerve stimuli but could still react to the adrenaline produced by the adrenal glands and secreted into the bloodstream. When the animal was exposed to cold, it was the adrenal glands that responded in order to warm the animal—otherwise it resorted to shivering. He found that the medullae in the adrenal glands participate in the function of the heart, in temperature control, and in many other basic activities.

Cannon went on to study "sympathetic nerves" throughout the body and showed that these nerves have almost identical functions to those of adrenaline from the adrenal medulla. Also, these nerves and the adrenal medulla work in collaboration to influence many organs. Both are crucial in local inflammation, including the control of blood flow to the inflamed part.

He established that the nervous system and the adrenal medulla have critical roles in our responses to emotion, pain, and exercise. As he put it: "These changes—the more rapid pulse, the deeper breathing, the increase of sugar in the blood, the secretion from the adrenal glands—were very diverse and seemed unrelated. Then, one wakeful night, the idea flashed through my mind that they could be nicely integrated if conceived as bodily preparations for supreme effort in flight or in fighting." In this "emergency" theory of the adrenal medulla, which explains a principal part of the body's responses to stress, Cannon described in 1914 what happens when "adrenaline runs in our veins."

We turn now to a Canadian experimental pathologist, Hans Selye. When I was a medical student at McGill University, many distinguished teachers inspired us. First, there was Stephen Leacock, whose humorous books, such as *Sunshine Sketches of a Little Town* and *Literary Lapses*, remain a delight. He had retired as Professor of Economics by the time I was at McGill, but he remained much in evidence on the campus and in the library. Wilder Penfield, the brilliant neurosurgeon and physiologist, lectured on epilepsy and sometimes interrupted his presentation to feign

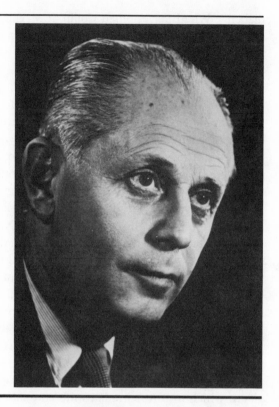

Hans Selye. A leading figure in establishing the association between stress and the body's endocrine response, Selye also studied the relationship between prolonged stress and disease.

some type of minor fit. Then there was Hans Selye. Even now, I have only to close my eyes to see a brilliant, restless, neat little man at the blackboard. To hold our attention, he drew simultaneously a cockerel with one hand and a hen with the other, all the while explaining the functions of the sex hormones at top speed.

Born in Vienna in 1907, Selye trained in Prague, Paris, Rome, and Baltimore before coming to McGill in 1932 to work in the Department of Biochemistry under the direction of James B. Collip, himself a fascinating investigator and the leading Canadian endocrinologist of his time. When a young professor in Alberta, Collip (a Toronto graduate) had been invited back to Toronto in 1921 to join in the discovery of insulin, following the preliminary experiments begun a few months before by Frederick Banting and Charles Best. It was Collip who first produced an extract of animal pancreas that was sufficiently pure and nontoxic to prove that insulin is invaluable in the treatment of human diabetes. When Selye joined Collip at McGill, the Department of Bio-chemistry was a hive of endocrinology research, devoted especially to the isolation and investigation of hormones of the parathyroid glands, the pituitary gland, and the ovaries.

In 1935, while working on sex hormones, Selye prepared an extract of ovaries and injected it into small animals. To his surprise, the adrenals were stimulated and the lymph nodes were atrophied—which could not be explained by any known hormone. He was elated. At the age of twenty-eight, he thought he had discovered a new hormone. But as weeks passed and he tried variations on the original experiment, he ob-tained the same result in too many ways. The cause could not be a new hormone. He eventually injected something entirely nonspecific, a di-lute solution of formalin; the adrenals and lymph nodes responded as they did after the ovarian extract. He was in despair. Then, after many days when he considered giving up, he dared to think what few people would have had the imagination or the courage to think: the response of the body to a nonspecific stimulus is of fundamental importance in medicine, and of far more significance than finding yet another hor-mone. Selye spent the rest of his life studying that response.

What emerged was that if an animal is persistently exposed to infec-tion, toxic substances, injury, cold, or fatigue, there is a critical long-term, protective response. The hypothalamus stimulates the pituitary gland, which in turn stimulates the adrenals. This process enables the animal to adapt to the threatening situation. If adaptation continues too long, it is no longer protective and may actually damage the animal. Among other complications, one feature of prolonged hormonal adap-tation is acute arthritis. Selye did not believe that this hormonal imbal-ance was the only cause—or even a prime cause—of arthritis, but he was convinced that it made animals more susceptible to arthritis.

Selye was years ahead of his time. It is not surprising that this revolu-tionary concept was rejected by most, and ridiculed by some, even though a number of perceptive scientists later traveled to Montreal to work under his direction. Years afterward Selye acknowledged that he might have made a mistake in referring to "stress-induced diseases" in-stead of to "diseases caused by failure of adaptation to noxious stimuli." One consequence of the name he originally chose was that the scientific world started viewing his findings in terms of emotional stress, which had not been the basis of his research. For many years Selye was revered by psychiatrists and psychologists, and either forgotten or spurned by

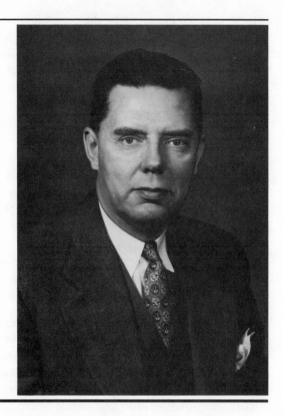

Philip Hench, Nobel Laureate. One of the pioneers of American rheumatology, Hench was codiscoverer of the therapeutic benefits of cortisone.

rheumatologists. Like most good science, though, what Selye did has been rediscovered and is currently the subject of intense research activity. Those involved in this work are amazed at how much Selye achieved at a time when many functions of endocrine glands were unknown.

At the same time Selye was doing his early work, researchers at the Mayo Clinic in Rochester, Minnesota, made a sensational discovery about the therapeutic benefits of cortisone. This account concerns two famous men, Philip Hench and Edward C. Kendall, who in 1950 shared (with Tadeus Reichstein of Switzerland) the Nobel Prize "for their discoveries relating to the hormones of the adrenal cortex, their structure and biological effects." Kendall's distinguished career as a chemist included the isolation, in 1914, of the active agent in the thyroid gland (thyroxine). Later, many laboratories investigated the adrenal cortex, which was then known to be the component of the adrenal gland that is essential to life. Several related adrenal hormones were identified, including compound E (cortisone), which was isolated by four different laboratories, including those of Reichstein and Kendall.

Philip Hench was born in Pittsburgh in 1896 and graduated in medicine from the University of Pittsburgh in 1920. The story goes that when he was a resident physician at the Mayo Clinic, intending to specialize in kidney diseases, he went on ward rounds with his chief, a nephrologist. At one bed the chief diagnosed osteoarthritis, while Hench, in an action unusual for those days, dared to contradict him and suggest a diagnosis of rheumatoid arthritis. On hearing this story, the renowned William Mayo became intrigued and asked Hench if he would like to become the Mayo Clinic's first specialist in arthritis. He was appointed to the staff on New Year's Day of 1926.

As early as 1929, Hench began to investigate the striking beneficial effects on arthritis of pregnancy and jaundice. Reviewing this work in 1949, he reached some encouraging conclusions:

> Even though the pathologic anatomy of rheumatoid arthritis is more or less irreversible, the pathologic physiology of the disease is potentially reversible, sometimes dramatically so. Within every rheumatoid patient corrective forces lie dormant, awaiting proper stimulation. Therefore, the disease is not necessarily a relentless condition for which no satisfactory method of control should be expected. In an attempt to reproduce the effects of jaundice or pregnancy, we and others used, more or less empirically, many agents and measures. In time we conjectured that the anti-rheumatic substance X might be an adrenal hormone.

Unkindly, it has been said that when Hench sought advice, Kendall simply took cortisone from the shelf—because it was there. Whether that is true or not, Hench selected a dose (which proved to be the correct one) and gave cortisone to fourteen patients. They all improved. He then organized a trial, comparing cortisone injections in some patients with cholesterol injections in others. The results were impressive, and at the time seemed even more dramatic. In movies (still available today), patients in the trial can be seen clambering slowly and painfully over obstacles, then, after treatment, leaping over the same obstacles. When the preliminary results were reported at medical meetings, even senior physicians stood on their chairs to cheer. But perhaps that remarkable beginning of cortisone treatment was too good to last.

Independent trials of an increasing range of cortisone-like drugs failed to show the same benefit, and the unpleasant side effects of this treatment became more apparent. It is difficult to be sure whether it was the side effects or the bitter disappointment that led to the unjustified hostility toward these drugs that is common today. The problem is that once rheumatoid arthritis is established, it is difficult to maintain improvement without continuing the treatment so long that side effects outweigh benefits. I have my own thoughts about the use of cortisone-like drugs in the treatment of rheumatoid arthritis, but to my regret I have never conducted a controlled trial of my own version of treatment; therefore I really have no right to comment. Nevertheless, let me report what forty patients with rheumatoid arthritis have taught me.

My view is that the correct time to start effective treatment is within weeks or months of the onset of symptoms—if necessary, before the diagnosis is firmly established. On modest doses of prednisone, given after frank discussion, a gratifying proportion of my patients have improved dramatically within days, in a way that could not be a placebo effect. Rheumatologists at a recent meeting in England voted in favor of a formal trial of prednisone used in this way, to determine whether it can succeed in nipping rheumatoid arthritis in the bud. My impression is that some patients recover fully, withdraw from therapy after a few weeks, and never relapse. But my experience tells me that after a year or more of symptoms it is too late to start this type of treatment. I cannot verify that statement as fact, but I mention it because it is important to appreciate that it may be possible early in the disease to prevent the progress of rheumatoid arthritis.

Today so many actions of this group of drugs are known that it is difficult to discern which is the most significant in treatment. It is tempting to cite the functions that suit any argument you wish to support. For example, in 1964 Max Wintrobe and his colleagues in Salt Lake City reported a highly relevant study. They recruited volunteers and used a standard technique to count the number of cells that appeared in an inflamed area of the skin. Their experiment demonstrated conclusively that when humans receive an injection of a cortisone-like drug, fewer cells pass through the lining of the blood vessels into the local tissue in response to an inflammatory stimulus. Recent evidence from New York indicates that the principal action of these drugs may be to diminish the endothelial cell production of molecules that adhere to white blood cells during local inflammation. But we now have so many established effects of cortisol, including those on actions within cells and between cells during inflammation, that no one can say with confidence why patients with arthritis do or do not get better.

Despite the drawbacks of cortisone-like drugs in some situations, and the understandable prejudice against them, this group of drugs is one of the most frequently prescribed of all medications. There are many indications for treatment, including striking benefit in several types of arthritis. To be impressed, one need only witness the initiation of treatment with prednisone for severe stiffness and pain due to polymyalgia rheumatica. A patient's symptoms can disappear within hours, as if by magic.

Within the past few years, several researchers have started to reinvestigate small animals with arthritis to assess the effects of the arthritis on the hypothalamus, pituitary, and adrenal glands. This work is undertaken knowing that the neuroendocrine system is far more complicated than originally envisaged, and taking advantage of the magnificent new techniques now available. For instance, Stafford Lightman (Professor of Neuroendocrinology), working with our group at Westminster Hospital, has demonstrated that the onset of experimental arthritis is associated with remarkable, seemingly inappropriate responses in the hypothalamus. And at the National Institutes of Health in Washington, D.C., Ronald Wilder and his colleagues have investigated strains of similar small animals and showed that differences in the function of the hypothalamus, pituitary, and adrenals between strains may influence their susceptibility to arthritis. In 1989 Jon Levine and his coworkers in San Francisco reported that after removal of the adrenal medulla in experimental animals (leaving the cortex intact), the animals became less susceptible to induced arthritis, and that susceptibility to arthritis was restored by infusing adrenaline (epinephrine).

The mechanisms we are investigating may not be the same as those proposed by Hans Selye, but we are all confirming that the hypothalamus, pituitary, and adrenals are probably important in determining when humans develop arthritis. This effect is certain to be complicated and to depend on many components of this highly sophisticated system rather than on any single hormone. However preliminary these results may be, research on the role of the neuroendocrine system in arthritis is definitely on the agenda to stay.

14

The Nervous System

The role of the nervous system in causing joint disease is one of the most intriguing aspects of rheumatology. I owe my own long-standing fascination with this subject to Angus McPherson, who was a colleague early in my career. Born in 1919, Angus studied medicine in Liverpool, joined the scientific staff of the Medical Research Council, and was appointed head of the neurophysiology unit at the Royal National Orthopaedic Hospital in London. When we met, he was concentrating on the neurophysiology of bones and joints. His knowledge of the field was profound, and his inquiring mind produced a stream of unorthodox ideas. We soon became firm friends. He taught me as much as he could about the frontiers of neurophysiology and the role of the nervous system in bone, periosteum, and synovium. We had endless discussions about the influence of the nervous system on arthritis, and soon I decided that this would be my principal research focus.

Through my involvement in the neurophysiology of bones and joints, I was invited in 1967 to organize a symposium on that subject for the Heberden Society. My task was to review all the clinical evidence that the nervous system is important in bones and joints. Angus spoke about viscero-somatic reflexes. A few weeks after the symposium, on the evening of May 3, we had a long telephone discussion about our future research together. Later that night, he died unexpectedly at the age of forty-seven. His death was a shocking loss for everyone, and the Medical Research Council followed its customary procedure of permanently closing down the unit in which he had worked. I concluded that it was no longer possible for me to study the neurophysiology of joints. For the next eighteen years I had to be content with teaching others that this was a fascinating subject waiting to be explored.

In Figure 18, I have simplified the anatomy of a typical section of the spinal cord. Because the brain thinks in terms of movements, not individual muscles, integrated messages are transmitted down the spinal cord to cells in the anterior part of the cord at the level controlling the muscles concerned. These messages are then transmitted by way of the nerve roots at the front of the spinal cord (anterior nerve roots), and from there they pass down the nerves to excite the muscles.

Sensations of pain, touch, position, and so on, coming from the periphery, are conveyed in sensory nerve fibers. Sensory messages indicating sensations enter the back of the spinal cord via the posterior nerve roots. In each of these roots is a bulge that contains the sensory nerve cells. Nerve fibers, which are highly specialized extensions of the sensory nerve cells, extend from the posterior nerve roots to the joints, skin, and other structures.

Figure 18 also shows the sympathetic nerves, which emerge from the

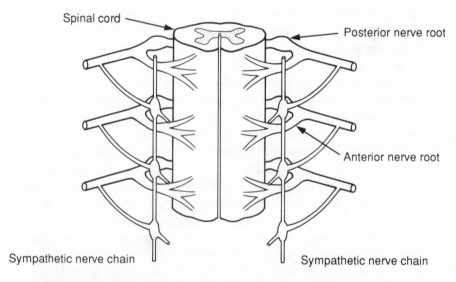

Figure 18 · A view of part of the spinal cord, seen from the front (anterior view).

motor and sensory nerves, just after the junction of the anterior and posterior nerve roots. The sympathetic nerves form two chains in front of the spinal cord that pass up and down the body, parallel to the cord.

In the second century, Galen very perceptively appreciated that inasmuch as every part of the body is connected to every other part of the body by nerves, they can all influence one another. Partly as a consequence of Galen's teaching, during the eighteenth and early nineteenth centuries it was widely believed by physicians, especially those in France, that the nervous system plays a role in most diseases. Even so, Julius Cohnheim strongly opposed the idea that the nervous system influenced inflammation, and for a long time this concept was the subject of controversy.

In 1874 it was demonstrated that stimulation of the sciatic nerve in a small animal resulted in local flushing due to dilation of the small blood vessels supplied by that nerve, much like the vessel dilation that takes place in inflammation. Shortly afterward, investigators showed the same response by stimulating posterior nerve roots. By the turn of the century we knew that this nerve root response was transmitted down the sensory nerves, in the direction opposite to the impulses conveying sensation. And it was soon found that small blood vessels have certain nerve fibers that make them dilate and other nerve fibers that make them constrict. When dilator nerve fibers were cut, small vessels became constricted and blood slowed to a trickle; hence any inflammatory response was reduced and recovery from injury delayed. Also, bacteria that had been injected locally were removed only slowly from the site. This type of nerve control is by conventional electrical impulses in sympathetic and other nerve fibers.

In the early part of this century A. Ninian Bruce of Edinburgh reported that the nerve reflexes which control blood vessels need not be mediated by the spinal cord. If a nerve has branches that supply some fibers to the skin and other fibers to a blood vessel, the nerve impulses can be transmitted between the skin and the blood vessel directly (by an axon reflex), short-circuiting the spinal cord.

By 1920 it was noticed that when the posterior nerve root was stimulated, the blood vessel delayed a few seconds before responding—much too long to represent a normal nerve impulse. Thirty years later it was suggested that an unidentified chemical slowly moved down the nerve fibers and made the blood vessels dilate. So one way that blood vessels are controlled is by a chemical secreted by the nerve fibers.

Earlier, in 1931, a new family of chemical substances known as neu-ropeptides had been identified. In 1953 Fred Lembeck discovered that one of the unknown chemicals that are formed in the posterior nerve roots is a neuropeptide (substance P). It has since been established that several neuropeptides originate in the cells of the posterior nerve roots, and from there the neuropeptides are transmitted down the nerve fibers. When they reach the joints, the neuropeptides are secreted by nerves in the synovium, bone, bone marrow, and periosteum. Among their many functions, neuropeptides can influence the dilation of blood vessels and the transport of fluid through the linings of small vessels. They can also modify the action of cells, especially those in the immune system.

No one has contributed more to our understanding of the association between the nervous system and arthritis than Jean-Martin Charcot, whom we have already met. Like Paul Ehrlich, Charcot was more than a genius; he was also an artist, with an artist's ability to observe shapes and patterns of movement. Moreover, he had an extraordinary capacity to remember visual images, thus enabling him to compare details in pa-tients with similar disorders. In his office, in lugubrious surroundings, one of his assistants would recount a patient's clinical history and phys-ical findings. Then, with the patient stripped before him, Charcot would make meticulous observations, paying particular attention to the move-ments. From all accounts he excelled as a clinician. He also embodied a medical approach that is sometimes forgotten today: it is usually of su-preme importance to observe patients in minute detail and to define the clinical problems accurately before proceeding to the laboratory.

Each year Charcot and his colleagues would concentrate on a different disorder. The period 1868 to 1869 was devoted to the joint abnormali-ties associated with tabes dorsalis, a disease in which syphilis damages the cells in the posterior nerve roots of the spinal cord. The result is a slowly progressive loss of the sensations of deep pain (in the joints, for example) and of position (leading to marked unsteadiness, especially in the legs). In advanced disease patients depend on vision to orient them-selves in space; they cannot tell automatically what their legs are doing.

Charcot knew that many people with tabes dorsalis developed a pe-culiar condition of one or more joints; and, unlike modern physicians, he had an almost unlimited number of untreated patients to investigate.

At the end of several months of detailed observation he reached the following conclusions:

> The clinical manifestations of the joint conditions are unique: There is a sudden onset of a generalized swelling of the limb; rapid changes occur in the surfaces of the joint which manifest themselves as crepitations that are often noticed a few days after the onset, their appearance being evidently determined by the duration of the spinal cord disease; and they usually precede the development of the characteristic motor incoordination of tabes. These disorders develop without apparent cause; they do not result exclusively, as has been claimed, from the distension undergone by the ligaments and capsules of the joints or from the awkward gaits characteristic of ataxic patients, because they are frequently located in the upper extremities or they may involve the shoulder or the elbow. Moreover, they can develop in patients who show no signs of motor incoordination.

Because this joint condition usually appeared early in the course of tabes, before the onset of motor incoordination, Charcot concluded that it was not caused simply by the loss of sensation. Drawing an incorrect parallel with pressure sores in paralyzed people, he made the extraordinary suggestion that the nerves might nourish the bones and joints so that, in disease, joint failure was due to lack of a "trophic factor" that nourished the local tissues.

For more than a hundred years Charcot's trophic factor was derided— on the basis of research that was far less satisfactory than Charcot had reported. Perhaps everyone was intolerant of a concept that had not yet been proved. Today Charcot would be delighted to look through our microscopes and see neuropeptides that have been formed in the cells of the posterior nerve roots and secreted in bone, in bone marrow, in periosteum, and in synovium—representing trophic factors such as Charcot might have imagined.

Isolated clinical reports suggest that local joint disease caused by rheumatoid arthritis or osteoarthritis, especially in the hand, is less severe when the affected limb has been paralyzed by a stroke or by poliomyelitis, or has lost the action of its sympathetic nerves as the result of surgery. But these reports represent only a few observations about widely differing clinical situations. And it is impossible to separate the effects of lack of physical use from lack of nerve function. This type of evidence alone is insufficient to build a reliable hypothesis on how the nervous system influences joint diseases.

More important evidence comes from poliomyelitis, a disease in which there is damage to the anterior cells in the spinal cord controlling the function of muscles. Studying this disease, colleagues at the Royal National Orthopaedic Hospital demonstrated a marked reduction in the frequency of osteoarthritis of the hip joint when there is local paralysis of the affected limb. Having observed the gait of many such people, I find it impossible to accept that a paralyzed joint is protected from physical damage. Hence, we know that local disease of the anterior part of the spinal cord prevents osteoarthritis, but in my opinion we do not yet understand the mechanism that leads to this prevention.

At the beginning of the present century, when interest in the microscopic appearance of osteoarthritis was intense, it was a matter of general discussion that changes in "Charcot's joints" and in osteoarthritis were remarkably similar. Still, it was never suggested seriously that osteoarthritis resulted from a disorder of the nervous system. But a sequel to Charcot's observations—a study of animals by a group in Cleveland, Ohio (reported in 1975)—showed that when the nerves of a knee joint were divided, the cells in the joint cartilage degenerated. This finding is particularly intriguing because nerve fibers have not been demonstrated in cartilage, yet it is the cartilage cells—the chondrocytes—that suffer first when the local nerve supply is abolished. One explanation, still to be investigated, is that Charcot's trophic factor (the neuropeptides secreted in bone) passes through the bone into the cartilage and nourishes the chondrocytes. If true, a local failure of the nerves in bone is conceivably a critical factor in osteoarthritis—a missing link in joint failure.

Now that neuropeptides and nerve fibers in bone can be investigated, we can turn to a long queue of questions that has accumulated as the result of clinical observations during the past hundred years. In many instances it is strongly suspected that the nervous system influences bone function.

When a bone is deformed or stressed mechanically, the bone's structure is modified and remodeled in conformity with physical principles—

and this response may prove to be controlled by the nervous system. In certain nervous diseases, fractured bones repair themselves at different rates. If the disease affects mainly the sensory fibers in nerves in the limbs, the fracture usually heals slowly and with difficulty; but if there is comparable loss of sensation in the limbs due to damage to the spinal cord or brain, the bone response is often excessive. To a clinician, it is as if the growth of bone were under the control of the nervous system. Furthermore, it has been speculated (but not proved) that nervous reflexes are involved in the loss of bone substance (osteoporosis) near inflamed joints, and possibly in the very common condition of generalized osteoporosis.

Before turning to the intriguing possibility that the nervous system may play a major role in inflammatory types of arthritis, let us look at two uncommon disorders and several that are common.

Reflex dystrophy is a strange condition in which the nervous system goes berserk for trivial reasons. In a typical example, a minor fracture of the wrist in an elderly woman—or for that matter, a young man—appears to be healing well. Then, unexpectedly, the shoulder, elbow, wrist, and hand of that limb become stiff and painful. At worst, the whole hand becomes an intensely painful, almost rigid, flipper, with virtually no useful function. On the few occasions when patients have volunteered for biopsy of a joint, the most striking feature has been disarray of cells in the synovium.

This involvement of one limb in a small proportion of patients is only the tip of the iceberg. Minor forms of the same condition are common, after a wide variety of trigger events. When obvious disease occurs in one limb, milder disease can usually be detected in its counterpart. Once established, this condition is extremely difficult to treat, not infrequently because of accompanying psychological factors. Sometimes striking improvement follows an injection to block the sympathetic nerves to the limb, supporting the belief that the nervous system has a significant role in this unpleasant disease.

I have already mentioned another unusual disease, hypertrophic pulmonary osteoarthropathy. HPOA is best known for its occasional association with lung cancer in older people, but it is now occurring in young people with cystic fibrosis. The characteristics of this uncommon condition are swelling of the ends of the fingers, arthritis of the finger joints or a few larger joints, and inflammation of the periosteum lining the bones in the limbs. There is appreciable widespread pain. Yet the

most remarkable feature is that the symptoms can be abolished immediately by certain procedures. After surgical removal of a lung tumor,
the joint pain often disappears on recovery from the anesthetic. The
same instant pain relief can follow cutting or injecting the vagus nerve,
which carries impulses from the lung first to the spinal cord and then to
the brain. Hence, we can speculate that this arthritis may be mediated
by the vagus nerve, probably by the hypothalamus, and possibly by the
sympathetic nerves to the joints and periosteum. Although less well established, it is quite possible that similar mechanisms contribute to
common conditions such as capsulitis of the shoulder, carpal tunnel
syndrome, and cervical and lumbar root compression.

To return to the quest for the causes of our key diseases, including
rheumatoid arthritis, it is instructive to consider the story of Leslie
Courtright, an allergist in San Francisco. In the 1960s he decided, for
family reasons, that he would like to investigate the causes of rheumatoid arthritis. So he approached a well-known rheumatologist, William
Kuzell, who arranged suitable laboratory accommodation and facilities.
Like many people coming new to a subject, Courtright had several fresh
ideas that had not occurred to anyone else. From them he selected one:
he wanted to determine whether the nervous system plays a part in inflammatory arthritis.

In experiments on small animals, Courtright divided the sciatic nerve
in one leg. After a period of recovery he induced the type of symmetrical,
experimental arthritis introduced by Carl Pearson (whom we met in
Chapter 4), in which dead tubercle bacilli are injected in the skin. Courtright's objective was to determine whether an arthritis that should be
symmetrical is influenced by the absence of nerve function in the ankle
joint on one side. Although the concept was brilliant, his results were
not conclusive. Courtright returned to his earlier work, unaware that his
contribution was to have major consequences.

In the 1980s the same approach was taken up again, first by Jon Levine and Allan Basbaum in San Francisco, then by Richard Rees and me
at Westminster Hospital. Rees and I found in our experimental model
that if the sciatic nerve is cut, the subsequent arthritis on that side is
always worse; and this local increase is not, as had been suggested, due
to lack of mobility. We and the San Francisco group found that unilateral
division of the posterior nerve roots severely aggravates the arthritis on
that side but reduces the arthritis on the opposite side. Blocking the
sympathetic nerves on one side has a marked, but more unpredictable

effect: sometimes it is worse on one side and sometimes on the other. The interpretation of all these results is difficult and intriguing.

A few years ago, Levine and Basbaum published an outstanding hypothesis with two main proposals: that neuropeptides secreted in joints may play a part in rheumatoid arthritis, and that the symmetry of arthritis may be determined by nervous reflexes. This latter proposal is in addition to the suggestion in Chapter 10 that the symmetry of joint disease could result from the symmetrical action of genes. Of course, there is no reason why both hypotheses should not be correct.

At least in our own experimental model, we have the provocative situation that if we block the nerve supply and deplete the neuropeptides in local joints, the ensuing arthritis is worse. Presumably, if the nervous system is intact, the arthritis is better; thus, the nervous system may have a powerful protective effect. My present research project is to determine whether this apparent protection against arthritis derives from an influence of the nervous system on the ability of cells and foreign substances to enter joints through the linings of small blood vessels—a possibility with obvious therapeutic implications. Whatever the details may prove to be, the nervous system is certainly capable of powerful influences on the onset, severity, and duration of inflammation in joints.

So far I have focused on the function of nerves and their connections with the spinal cord. We know far more about them, because it is much easier to investigate their relatively simple actions than it is to study the brain and the mind. But there is more than a suspicion that the brain may have a supervisory role in the immune system, inflammation, and arthritis. When describing the immune system and its responses in Chapter 2, I gave the impression that its complicated means of communicating and handling foreign and abnormal substances has no central control, no headquarters. But we have mounting, not absolute, evidence that the immune system is less autonomous in its actions than was once believed, and that the brain and the hypothalamus are active in a supervisory role. As a compelling example, a scientific study was conducted by the Medical Research Council in London on whether hypnosis affects inflammation upon injection of dead tubercle bacilli into the skin (the Mantoux test, which originated from the work of Robert Koch). After an experienced hypnotist had made an appropriate suggestion to the subject, the local blood vessels did not dilate following the injection, and no fluid came to the site so there was no local swelling. Yet skin biopsies revealed that cells arrived in expected numbers. Hypnosis had clearly prevented part of the expected inflammatory response.

The distinguished French physiologist Claude Bernard (1813–1878) was the first to appreciate the importance of physiological adaptation to psychological and social problems in the causation of disease. His concept was that disease often results from the nervous system's inappropriate reaction to stress. In his view, tissues are pressed beyond their limits, and this leads not only to symptoms but sometimes to tissue destruction. Bernard was followed by Cannon, Selye, and others who studied how emotion and stress affect adrenal hormones, nerves, blood vessels, and the immune system. It is necessary, however, to underline that because they were investigating small animals all of these researchers wrote about simple psychological mechanisms.

To put the function of the nervous system on a higher plane, consider the work of a brilliant New York physician and neurophysiologist, Harold Wolff (whom I had the pleasure of meeting while I was a student). He felt strongly that stress could not be defined solely in terms of a person's surroundings, but must also include the person's *perception* of those surroundings. He saw no line of demarcation between a response to local physical injury and a complicated psychological defense:

> A multitude of protective and compensatory attitudes may serve to carry an individual through a crisis, even in the absence of feelings of anxiety. For example, unacceptable facts, situations, or conflicts, may be repressed, forgotten, denied, misrepresented, pretended to be other than they are, made light of, joked, or clowned about . . . These and many other defensive devices and combinations, once established, maintained, and elaborated in a socially acceptable way, may become permanent components of personality. However, should the load become too great, or too long-lasting, such attitudinal defenses may break down or be supplemented by more primitive devices.
>
> Since all these responses relevant to disease are integrated at the highest functional level of the brain, one naturally asks whether this organ itself may be damaged as a consequence of improper interaction between organism and environment, more particularly, faulty interaction between human creatures. There is much to indicate that this is so.

Without doubt, when we consider hormones and nerves, we must think about the response of the whole person. The neuroendocrine system, the nervous system, and psychological and social factors work together in our lives—in ways far more complicated than the concepts of stress derived from experiments on small animals. Although the precise mechanisms are not yet understood, it is anticipated that these processes will prove to be extremely important in determining whether we are subject to several diseases, including arthritis, and the time at which we are most susceptible.

15

Personality, Emotions, and Pain

No illness has the same consequences for everyone, because we are all individuals—with our own experiences, hopes and fears, families, jobs, communities, and relationships with society. Hence, not all science takes place in laboratories or at the bedside. We have learned much, and have far more to learn, from psychologists, psychiatrists, social workers, clinicians, and others in the social sciences. From this immense topic I have elected to concentrate on three items: the universal process of reporting symptoms such as pain, emotionally threatening events before the onset of rheumatoid arthritis, and reactions after the onset of disease.

Everyone has pain from time to time, and all of us find life difficult once in a while. Physical disease, social problems, and psychological factors inevitably overlap. Few people experience pain due exclusively to psychological problems without an element of physical abnormality; and few suffer arthritis or other diseases without some personal issues. Thus, we must ask, "How is pain modified by physiological or psychological mechanisms; and which factors influence whether, and how, people complain about their pain?"

First is the physiological fact that pain impulses, after traveling in the sensory fibers to reach the posterior nerve roots and then the spinal cord, enter a local pool of cells in the spinal cord that integrates the nerve impulses from various sources. As a consequence, a pain may be enhanced or diminished by something that happens in another part of the body. Or two mild sources of pain in the same region may supplement each other and result in a more severe pain, with a distribution unlike that of either constituent pain on its own. In this way a heart pain and a joint pain may combine to produce a pain of an entirely different character.

Psychological factors can also aggravate or diminish the sensation of pain. A person who is bored, lonely, and depressed, and who sits brooding over a swollen foot, will be certain to feel far more pain than a soldier who suffers a severe leg wound at the height of battle.

Natural substances, endorphins, can reduce the sensation of pain; but despite claims by enthusiasts, so far we do not know enough about their function to apply this knowledge effectively in treatment.

The psychological perception of pain depends on a lifetime of experiences. It is strongly affected by cultural differences, by childhood training, by inbuilt sensitivities, by varying capacities to cope, and so on; and there is good evidence that neurotic behavior in childhood may be followed by neurotic behavior as an adult. Some patients genuinely suffer more severe pain because they grew up in an atmosphere where pain was the best means of attracting the attention that most children enjoy as an expression of affection.

Pain is also aggravated or prolonged by the full range of psychological difficulties experienced as an adult. Depression, anxiety, frustration, grief, family strife, sexual difficulties, alcohol or drug abuse, the dreariness of long winters bereft of sunlight, unresolved anger, or personal gain may all play a part, as do fundamental factors such as sexuality, aggression, or dependency.

Reporting pain to someone can be viewed as a somewhat separate process, and it is as complicated as the individual's perception of his or her own pain. Founded on a lifetime experience of bringing problems to the attention of other people, this special form of education starts at birth and continues throughout the critical first year. After that come the years of running to mummy or daddy for comfort. This background of learned behavior strongly influences when an individual is likely to seek advice about a persistent pain, and from whom: physician, priest, naturopath, faith healer, pharmacist, spouse, relative, or neighbor.

Patients frequently consult a physician hoping for psychological help, but not liking to ask. They may present nice, respectable symptoms with one hand, while keeping the real problems behind their back in the other hand. Only after they learn to trust the physician do they signal that they might be willing to discuss the hidden issues.

Next is the response of the person whose help you are seeking. For example, you may have had a parent who did not comfort you, but instead scolded and possibly struck you. How you react to a reception that you perceive as antagonistic is largely based on how your complaints have been received from early childhood. Many patients dislike physicians, or blame them for the pains they have had in the past; the busy physician who does not listen sympathetically may induce hostile feelings against all physicians to whom the patient may complain in the future. As a result, it is not unusual for a patient consulting a physician for the first time to give the impression that he has not come to talk about his pain so much as to complain about the last physician he consulted.

Then there is the complex process of self-diagnosis. In the past, individuals either made up their own mind or sought advice from books or friends. In this age of communication, they are influenced by the full force of the media, including regular comments on illness in newspapers, magazines, books, and on radio and television. This spread of information is excellent in many ways, leading as it does to early requests for medical advice and better understanding of disease. It is also a powerful mechanism for sweeping away ignorance and prejudice. For example, it would be beneficial if it were widely known that "rheumatism" denotes little more than a misconception of the ancient Greeks. How much better it would be if people knew more about arthritis, because today most individuals, once they have pain in two or more joints, readily assume that they have rheumatoid arthritis and will be crippled and confined to a wheelchair within two years. They have nightmares in which they see themselves as misshapen, asexual, and unable to work, love, or look after their families.

Improved communication is not totally beneficial, however. In addition to its many advantages, some misconceptions become more firmly entrenched. Indeed, new concepts of disease may undergo trial by media before physicians have enough scientific evidence on which to base reliable conclusions. Present-day well-informed patients consult physicians not only with complex problems hidden behind their back, but sometimes with confident views about their diagnosis and treatment, all protected by elaborate defenses to prevent the physician from venturing an opinion.

These general principles, which I have summarized in terms of complaints about pain, apply to many other symptoms and to many disorders. My purpose has been to introduce a major human problem that results in disability in a substantial proportion of the population. This condition, while in the mind of the public associated with joint diseases, is not principally the result of arthritis as understood by physicians. The condition lacks a suitable name and is generally called rheumatism, but the pain it causes is troublesome and usually entirely genuine. Sufferers are not exaggerating.

When, in a social gathering, talk turns to "rheumatism" and "arthritis," as it often does, a remarkable number of people begin animated discussions about their own symptoms. They are seldom the people who have definite diagnoses of arthritis or other physical disorders, because those people have thought about their condition and have either come to terms with it or suppressed their inner feelings. Rather, I am referring to the immense group of men and women who have diagnosed *themselves* as having "rheumatism" or "arthritis," either on their own or with assistance from their physicians. It is difficult to calculate the size of this group from the evidence available, but my estimate would be about one-quarter of adults of middle age or older—and many younger people as well. For most of them their ailment is little more than cause for comment, like talking about the weather, but for others it is more serious; and, sadly, there is a substantial number for whom "rheumatism" and "arthritis" have become established as parts of their patterns of behavior.

As a background to their complaints, a high proportion in this group have previously had minor injuries or niggling physical disorders, or currently have slight wearing of joints or other conditions. But, by definition, their disabilities and complaints far exceed their physical abnormalities. Their difficulties are principally psychological and stem from the whole range of factors that influence whether people complain of pain.

It is not by accident that we use terms such as "working one's fingers to the bone," "a back-breaking job," "the care of the world on one's shoulders," or "a pain in the neck." The stresses and strains of life, depression, grief, anxiety, frustration, anger, and so on are rejected as self-diagnoses because it is more acceptable to have "rheumatism" or "arthritis." Thus, for example, one-third of people with depression severe enough to require psychiatric advice have previously consulted someone else about their physical aches and pains.

Most individuals live in harmony with their rheumatic complaints. But for many people there are serious disadvantages. After a few years the concept of "rheumatism" may be so deeply embedded that it is difficult for a physician, or anyone else, to suggest an alternative explanation for the symptoms; and the substitution of one diagnosis for another may make it impossible for individuals to face up to treatment or other measures to combat the real problems. At worse, the "rheumatism" or "arthritis" eventually dominates the lives of the sufferers and their families. Other physical diagnoses may be added. Ultimately the defenses are so elaborate that no one can question the self-diagnosis or institute effective help. We are obliged to collude and to sympathize.

The "rheumatism" must also be treated. At first a hairdo or a new hat may suffice (and there is nothing wrong with that), but next the sufferer may resort to nature cures, massage, herbal remedies, diets, tablets, faith healing, homeopathy, chiropractic, osteopathy, and visits to physicians—all of which may be effective and beneficial, but almost inevitably expensive. Indeed, we are talking about a multibillion-dollar business.

Rheumatologists with a special interest in the psychological aspects of pain have always been well acquainted with a large group of patients who complain of ill-defined, widespread, mild-to-moderate pain associated with multiple points of tenderness. These symptoms stem from many psychological issues, often deep-rooted and difficult to treat. A few years ago it was proposed that these symptoms had a physical basis; the ailment was named the "fibromyalgia syndrome," which means pain in the connective tissues and muscles. Although scientific evidence to support the physical component is still slender, the consequence has been an epidemic of fibromyalgia throughout the world. Psychologists have recently studied people with severe fibromyalgia and confirmed that most of them have psychological problems, the nature of which varies from individual to individual. While some physicians and psychologists believe that a diagnosis such as "fibromyalgia" is beneficial because it is kinder and more acceptable than, say, "depression," others rightly point out that once such a diagnosis is made, the prospects of assisting with the psychological problems may be sharply diminished.

A further problem is highlighted in a recent random survey of over a thousand adults in an English population. Fifty-five percent had experienced pain during the previous month. As many as 16 percent had had symptoms characteristic of fibromyalgia during that period, which suggests that the disease as it is encountered by physicians may be determined at least as much by the factors that prompt patients to seek advice as by the initial causes of the symptoms.

In another group of patients the dominant complaint is prolonged, disabling fatigue, associated with widespread discomfort, disturbances of sleep, or unusual forms of depression. Recently, it has been proposed that this condition results from a persistent viral infection, and it has been called "postviral fatigue syndrome" (also known as "myalgic encephalomyelitis" or "ME"). By definition, it follows an acute viral infection. As with fibromyalgia, the evidence that this syndrome has a physical cause is incomplete and difficult to prove, thus leading to different interpretations by experts in the field. Some physicians say that ME is a physical disease; others say it is not; most are awaiting further evidence. What is not in dispute is that a wide range of psychological disorders is common among some people with ME. Also, this diagnosis has attracted large numbers of people who do not have ME. Furthermore, newly formed ME societies exhibit group hostility toward physicians who suggest that psychological factors are important. Whether or not a physician accepts the physical basis of this syndrome, it has become virtually impossible to question a perceived diagnosis of myalgic encephalomyelitis.

Given the many types of arthritis, the diseases that can masquerade as arthritis, the worn joints, sprains, and other physical disorders, and all the psychological and social factors that lead people to seek medical help, it is not surprising that a first consultation with a physician may be confusing for both patient and doctor. As a consequence, physicians must be prepared to make a balanced assessment of the psychological, social, and physical issues, and above all be prepared to listen.

Fortunately, the diagnosis of arthritis and other physical disease is usually comparatively straightforward for an experienced physician. Psychological issues present more difficulty. The interview may resemble the games two people play. The patient comes having selected pieces of information that he or she considers to be relevant and respectable, while concealing other information; at the same time, the physician may make the diagnosis and then have to consider whether it is expedient to tell the patient what it is. Much of the consultation may consist largely of the two players assessing each other.

One of the physician's main objectives is to determine why the patient has come, and what he or she should know—or would like to know. If the issue is physical diagnosis, or methods of pain relief, or whether the patient is likely to become crippled, the answer may be simple and the patient's relief may be obvious. Similarly, if the patient is plucking up the courage to ask about an emotional problem, the solution may not be simple, but at least the essential issue has been defined.

The constant trap is a diagnosis that the patient finds intolerable. Few people presenting with physical symptoms can accept a diagnosis of depression; and physicians know how traumatic it may be if they tell someone who has had "rheumatism" or "arthritis" for several years that it is not true and that he or she does not have arthritis. Of course, some patients are delighted and greatly relieved, but many immediately become angry and make it clear that they will consult someone else in the future. A common way of avoiding such fury is to adopt a middle course. It may be possible to assist with some of the patient's hidden problems without mentioning the intolerable subject of diagnosis. Sometimes one can listen to the causes of frustration and anger, arrange interim treatment, or even give an antidepressant with the patient's consent—with the objective of returning to more delicate issues at a later date.

To illustrate some of these difficulties, let me recount how ten people presented their symptoms.

As an elementary example, I was consulted by a young woman who complained of lumbar backache. When I examined her, she bent over and touched the floor with twice the speed of a normal person, as if to say in body language, "Surely, you can see that this is not my real problem." During the second interview she told me of an experience when, years before, she had arrived in a small town in South Africa and discovered that she might have contracted an embarrassing disease that required urgent treatment. At first she could not decide what to do, but after three days of anxiety she consulted a physician and told him that she had backache, a condition that she had had before. If he was a nice, kind physician, she would ask about her real difficulty. Fortunately, he was a nice, kind physician; she did have the condition she was worried about, and she was treated successfully. After being offered that story, I had no difficulty in learning her true reason for seeing me. The backache was forgotten.

A fifty-year-old actress sprained a finger joint. Because it was still swollen and uncomfortable after nine months—which is not unusual— she concluded that she had arthritis. Her nights became disturbed by repeated nightmares in which she had rheumatoid arthritis and was crippled. She gradually developed more widespread symptoms, which seemed to confirm her anxiety. The problem was resolved by an unambiguous diagnosis of a sprain and by reassurance that she would soon recover satisfactorily.

A painter, aged twenty, had low lumbar backache related to a mild disc disorder; and he was unable to work for several months. The difficult issue for me as physician was to determine why, apart from the man's occupation, his pain was continuing much longer than expected. When the patient was given an opportunity to talk, he poured out his complicated feelings about his homosexuality.

A lecturer, thirty years old, had troublesome intermittent pain in the neck related to a minor condition of the local ligaments. It was not obvious why the pain was so troublesome, however, until I asked her two questions. In response to "Do you relate your pain to any particular person?" she said "Yes," and to "If you had ten minutes to make your problem worse, how would you set about it?" she replied, "I would have a row with my boss." The truth was that her conditions at home and at work were intolerable. After she had been encouraged to ventilate her problems, she decided to resign from her job and to return to her hometown. Her neck pain then subsided and she had no further trouble.

By contrast, a woman of thirty-five complained of vague pains, which she was reluctant to define clearly. Before she married she had had a good, well-paid job. Now she had a pleasant home and four children, one of whom was physically disabled and mentally subnormal but living with the family. Her husband could never come to terms with the unfortunate child: he drank, he stayed out late; and sometimes he hit his wife. Without doubt her "arthritis" was an important symbol for her—a protest against her insoluble situation. She could not have tolerated being told that she did not have arthritis, nor did she particularly want to talk about it. A social worker was doing everything possible, so all I could do was listen at length to her real problems and tell her that her physical condition was mild and likely to settle spontaneously. She had not expected anything more.

A young man saw me because he had been unable to work for a year following a mild sprain of a toe joint. As I listened to his story, I soon appreciated that he was not really interested in his toe. He kept telling me about the dreadful young surgeon whom he had seen at a nearby hospital after he was injured. According to my patient's account, the surgeon was incompetent: he did not make the correct diagnosis; he was rude; and he discharged him too soon. The patient was obviously seeing me because of a misplaced belief that I would help him to get revenge. It was only necessary for me to listen sympathetically and say nothing. The next day he went back to work.

A thirty-year-old woman had an ill-defined pain in one thigh. She had been a delicate child, suffering repeated attacks of unexplained abdominal pain. She was often absent from school. At fourteen she was diagnosed as having chronic anxiety which resulted in vague symptoms in different parts of her body. There was a history of childhood sexual abuse, for which she had received counseling. When examination and investigation were negative, and I suggested that the thigh pain was another symptom of her anxiety, she replied, "Well, if it's only my anxiety again, I know how to deal with that." No doubt she subsequently developed different symptoms in other parts of her body and sought advice elsewhere.

A housewife of sixty was beset by general aches and pains. After a while friends noticed that she had become forgetful and less well organized. Then she experienced delusions at night, seeing small creatures on the wall. She had a thyroid deficiency. After two weeks of hormone therapy with thyroxine, she made a full recovery.

A company director, aged seventy, slowly developed a sense of discomfort and stiffness. His symptoms were mild, and at first they occurred only occasionally. Gradually they became worse, particularly at night. Both shoulders were stiff and he experienced discomfort in the neck and back. Sometimes his hips were painful or it was difficult to turn over in bed. He decided that he was just old and neurotic, and that he had better retire from work and give up playing golf. At first he refused to see a physician because he did not want to make a fuss. He had polymyalgia rheumatica and recovered immediately when treated with prednisone.

A secretary aged twenty-three complained of discomfort around the chest, with occasional bouts of discomfort in the neck or thighs. Sometimes one thigh was uncomfortable as she put weight on it; then, the following week, she might have discomfort in the opposite thigh. Blood tests and x-rays were normal, and her physician could not make a diagnosis. People thought she was neurotic. In the absence of a diagnosis, she became anxious and mildly depressed. The correct diagnosis was ankylosing spondylitis. After taking tablets to reduce the inflammation in her spine, her symptoms largely disappeared.

We turn now to an old question concerning the causes of arthritis; almost from the time that rheumatoid arthritis was defined as a disease, some have suggested that it might result from psychological stress. Although this view has been unpopular during the past forty years, it has recently reappeared as an issue that must be taken into account.

In 1907 T. S. P. Strangeways (who later founded the Strangeways Laboratory) and J. B. Burt reviewed the available anecdotal evidence concerning the causes of rheumatoid arthritis. They reported that before the onset of their disease, patients often passed through a period of anxiety or strain. Several previous authors had mentioned worry, anxiety, depression, or shock as causes of the disease. Strangeways and Burt recorded three representative cases:

- A man developed rheumatoid arthritis following the prolonged bursting of shells during a siege.
- A woman had nursed her mother and her four sisters, all of whom died of tuberculosis, shortly before she had an onset of rheumatoid arthritis.
- A woman fifty years of age found a thief stealing a money box containing all her wealth. She ran after him for four miles but failed to catch him. A few weeks later she developed rheumatoid arthritis.

After that early document, doctors occasionally studied the possibility that psychological factors make people susceptible to rheumatoid arthritis; but almost all of the studies were criticized for the serious defect that the patients could not report accurately on what had happened to them several years before. So at Westminster Hospital we decided in 1976 to reinvestigate this subject by a team approach. My responsibility was to assess women who had had symptoms of rheumatoid arthritis for less than twelve months. I determined the provisional diagnosis at that time and the definitive diagnosis two years later. After my first examination all the women were interviewed by the consultant psychiatrist working in the rheumatology department. In a second study, they were seen by a research psychologist. In all we assessed over fifty patients. The controls were volunteers drawn from the list of a general practitioner, and they were matched by age to the nearest year.

Particularly interesting to me were the one-third of these women who had swollen, stiff, and painful fingers, exactly like rheumatoid arthritis, who then recovered and did not develop lasting disease. Many of them had evidence of emotional stress and anxiety when first seen. The clinical picture was like a form of rheumatoid arthritis that had failed to become established; it appeared to have a clear relation to stress or persistent anxiety.

Of the women who developed undoubtedly true rheumatoid arthritis, 50 percent had undergone emotionally threatening life events, compared with 15 percent of the controls. In the three months before the onset of their symptoms, most of the rheumatoid patients had had experiences that constituted moderate or considerable long-term emotional threats to their lives.

One difficulty with this type of investigation was that at the time of assessment the patients already had a disease that they had every reason to dislike. Therefore, they looked back with suspicion at anything that preceded it and might be held responsible. As we provided prolonged medical care for these women after our initial evaluation, however, we were confident that the events they reported were genuinely related to the onset of their rheumatoid arthritis.

As a final topic, we will consider a few of the psychological issues that accompany the onset of arthritis and the all-important relationship between patient and physician.

Soon after I graduated in medicine, I read an autobiography that made a lasting impression on me. It started with the life of a young undergraduate at Oxford. In her early university days, life revolved around boat races, lawns, spires, May balls, and her hopes and dreams for the future. Then, at the age of nineteen, she suffered a sudden onset of arthritis, first in one knee and then elsewhere. Her hopes were destroyed; most of her dreams vanished. What struck me forcibly was that she consulted several physicians; one after another, they looked away because they could not face a beautiful young woman whom they were unable to help. No professional person gave her the support and advice she needed so desperately. Her book confirmed for me that in such circumstances it is essential to establish mutual trust.

Although at the beginning of a potentially persistent illness, patient and physician always hope for the best, it is also necessary to plan for the worst. They must lay the foundations for a long-term relationship, as demanding for the physician as any he or she is likely to experience. From the outset there is a risk that the easy options in treatment and management may not succeed, thus leading to disastrous collapse of the patient's confidence. Truth and frank discussion are essential. The art is to judge how much the patient wishes to know, and then to provide that advice and information—no more and no less. Total management of a patient's care and all the details of the treatment given will depend on the nature of the relationship between patient and physician. If the physician is unaware of the psychological and social issues involved and the relationship is poor, the patient will require more drug therapy than may be wise—and will certainly not fare as well.

The most taxing period in the course of a disease such as rheumatoid arthritis is the first two years after the onset of symptoms. It is not only a time of massive adjustment, it is also by far the best opportunity to reverse the disease by effective treatment and to prevent it from becoming established. How patients react emotionally at the onset of arthritis depends largely on their experiences throughout life and their perceptions of joint diseases. Some react superbly from the beginning and readily become adjusted to their new situation. Others succumb too easily and adopt a passive response, sometimes even withdrawing from life. Still others deny what is happening and refuse all help offered to them, as if to accept would be a sign of weakness. A few work twice as hard as usual to prove to themselves that they do not have arthritis. We also need to consider whether patients are troubled by emotionally threatening life events that occurred before the onset of their disease, for help with the consequences of these harrowing experiences often assists the patients in their adjustment to arthritis.

While the person with arthritis may have access to all sorts of suitable advice, there are special difficulties for the spouse, who suffers much of the anguish and may receive no advice at all. The children of the patient also have special problems: although they usually are remarkably adaptable and understanding, they are peculiarly vulnerable. The onset of arthritis in a parent obviously can be extremely disturbing and threatening for the children in the family. Then there are friends and relatives who know little about arthritis and are confused by their inability to help. With the best of intentions, in their embarrassment they may make inappropriate comments and suggest remedies they would never consider for themselves. At the same time, they yearn to give genuine help.

For those with early arthritis, admission to a hospital often has two remarkable effects. First, going to bed and throwing off the stresses and responsibilities of everyday life, like returning to the cradle, may bring about dramatic relief of pain and inflammation within hours. This phenomenon is as striking as the response to cortisone-like drugs, but it has never been investigated with the same intensity. Second, patients who are floundering in their emotional response to this new enemy have time to reflect and opportunity to ask questions. From then on they may adopt totally different attitudes, such as a willingness to accept help without resenting the need to do so.

In the early months of the disease, emotional stress is a major difficulty. Far too many people struggle on (usually of necessity) against pain and fatigue when they should accept the need for rest and mental relaxation. Although this is not a solution for most, a few wealthy people with early arthritis arrange to go beachcombing and otherwise relax in warm and congenial places, after which they return home remarkably improved.

The relationship of physician, patient, and family is undoubtedly of paramount importance during the critical first two years of arthritis. To illustrate some of these issues, let me recount the clinical problems presented by six representative patients.

Early in my career I saw a woman in her late twenties who was grievously disabled by arthritis. Over the course of several interviews, she told me the truth about her original illness. She had had a lonely, protected childhood. As she approached her fourteenth birthday, arrangements were made for her to become an apprentice hairdresser. On the morning she was due to start work, she awoke with pain in all of her joints, which proved to be due to rheumatoid arthritis. Years afterward she remembered vividly her deep sense of relief as she sank back into the pillows, realizing that she would not have to face the outside world. As her arthritis became worse, she remained in bed, never leaving the house—for thirteen years. She eventually developed an acute disorder of the thyroid gland and mercifully was admitted to a hospital, by then unable to walk. After intensive rehabilitation, she learned to walk again, to live independently, and to drive a car. And she finally went out to work. I have never known anyone with more courage.

After a disturbed, neurotic childhood, a young woman sought refuge in marriage. The outcome was a new family deprived of love, and more neurotic children. She then developed arthritis, which progressed rapidly and resulted in apparently unnecessary deformity of the legs. We were faced with a woman who used her arthritis as an immature means of attracting attention and dominating her ill-tempered family. Her bewildered husband responded by undermining her confidence with excessive sympathy, instead of supporting a positive and courageous approach to independence. All of our attempts to correct her deformities failed. Trapped in this pattern of behavior, she sank beneath the waves. Her hatred of her pain and of her arthritis steadily increased until, tragically, they destroyed her life and her family.

A forty-year-old manicurist had had rheumatoid arthritis for seven years. Her hands were of immense emotional importance to her, and when they became mildly swollen and deformed, she sat on them or wore gloves to hide them. She tried all kinds of treatments, orthodox and unorthodox, but her hands still looked abnormal. When first I saw her, she had totally unrealistic hopes for surgery and wanted to know whether she could have operations to make her hands look normal. It was a difficult decision because the prime purpose of such surgery is to improve function rather than appearance. The orthopedic surgeon agreed to operate, but only after laying out clear objectives and insisting that she adopt a more reasonable expectation of what might be achieved.

A man of thirty had arthritis and lost his job as a printer. Each time he applied for a job the prospective employer rejected him, usually because he did not understand arthritis and was afraid to take the risk of recruiting someone who might become seriously disabled. When I first saw the man, he had been unemployed for three years. Throughout that time he had attended the clinic regularly for pain pills. After I briefed the hospital's rehabilitation officer, he went with the patient to negotiate a suitable job within the printing trade. After that he required no time off from work and quickly regained his confidence and self-respect. When I saw him six months later and asked about pills for his pain, he replied, "What pain?"

Soon afterward, I was troubled by the care of a distressed and poor young woman whose husband had left her. The medical problem was that she had severe, generalized arthritis of both hands. I tried every treatment I could imagine, but she only got worse. At last someone whispered to me that she had four children under the age of six; and since she had no washing machine, she was wringing all her laundry by hand. After we bought her a washing machine with special funds, her hands began to improve; subsequently, she continued to do well.

A pleasant woman in her late fifties consulted me. Seven years before, her husband had died suddenly. Within weeks she developed arthritis. Fortunately, the initial episode settled down and her arthritis caused little trouble most of the time. But whenever a friend or relative died, her joints became painful and swollen for several weeks. After prolonged discussion, the patient and I decided that instead of drug therapy, it would be better for her to seek counseling for her unresolved grief. When I saw her two years later, she was doing extremely well.

16

Populations and Families

Although physicians are primarily interested and involved in the care of individuals, medical science has recognized since its earliest beginnings that much can be learned from studying families and groups of people in communities. This approach, called epidemiology, is formally described as "the study of diseases and their characteristics within defined populations." During many investigations of diseases of obscure or unknown origin, epidemiology has supplied the foundation on which other work could build. As examples, we have already discussed the impact of contagion and the advantages of quarantine, which were well established several centuries before germs were known to cause disease.

Without the solid basis contributed by epidemiology, few problems in the study of arthritis could have been solved and few advances could have been made in understanding joint diseases. So far in this book, I have drawn heavily on information provided by epidemiological research, especially the distribution of different types of arthritis—in many countries, between the sexes, and at different ages. Yet I have held in reserve other important observations so that I can illustrate some of the techniques involved in studies of this sort.

One of the earliest epidemiological investigations of arthritis was during the late fifth and early fourth century B.C., when the Greek physician Hippocrates initiated an inquiry into the distribution of gout in the community. Later investigations of communities, notably in the eighteenth century by William Heberden the Elder (whom we met in Chapter 10), had limited significance; for little progress could be made until diseases

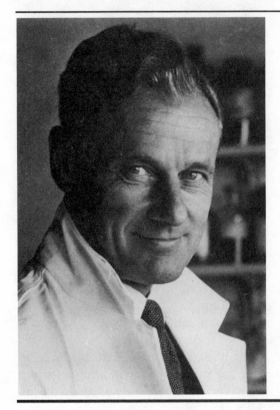

Jonas Kellgren. After World War II, Kellgren was unsurpassed in establishing modern arthritis research, including the use of epidemiological techniques in studying families and populations.

such as rheumatoid arthritis and osteoarthritis had been identified and widely accepted. The earliest modern epidemiological study in this field, published in 1921, was based on the frequency of rheumatic diseases in the workplace. Then, in 1928, the founding of the International League Against Rheumatism led to several epidemiological surveys, notably in Russia, Sweden, Germany, and Scotland. But it was not until after World War II that epidemiological investigations of arthritis began on a large scale, led by small groups of rheumatologists in the United States, Finland, the Netherlands, and England.

Looking back at that early research, most physicians today recognize the outstanding contributions of Jonas Kellgren to the epidemiology of arthritis. In 1947 Kellgren served as Director of the Rheumatism Research Centre in Manchester and later was appointed to England's first professorial chair of rheumatology. He and his close colleague, John

Lawrence, were pioneers in this type of research. At the time they began their work, statistics were being collected from hospitals, from work incapacity certificates, from general practitioners' lists, and from other sources, but none of these had provided a reliable guide to the frequency of different types of arthritis. Questionnaires were also unreliable because of the low completion rate. So Kellgren and Lawrence decided to organize teams and to go out among the people.

Having obtained a mobile trailer with clinical, laboratory, and x-ray facilities, they set out to examine individuals in their own communities. They soon found that it was too expensive and time-consuming to achieve their ideal of selecting people completely at random. Compromise was essential. Often their objective was achieved by examining clusters of people living in areas surrounding geographic points that had been chosen at random. It became apparent that there could be no shortcuts in the assessment of individuals. There was no possibility of simply taking blood samples and x-rays, and neglecting clinical examination, because there proved to be poor correlation between rheumatoid factor in the blood, x-ray results, and clinical findings.

By the time the work of Kellgren and Lawrence was well under way, definitions of diseases and diagnostic criteria had become a matter of worldwide cooperation. International conferences were held in Maryland (1957), in Rome (1961), and in New York (1966). Formal surveys could then be conducted everywhere in the world and the results could be compared. Encouraged by early results, epidemiologists mounted more expensive and more elaborate investigations. In the Netherlands they performed a national survey of sixty-eight municipalities. And a few years later in the United States nineteen hundred areas were surveyed by geographic location and population density.

Other surveys were longitudinal in time, with selected populations examined on several occasions. Some studies were repeated for a year—with the object of distinguishing between transient and persistent diseases. In a few surveys, the same people were reinvestigated every year, or every five years. Several countries organized major prospective surveys in which thousands of representative people were questioned and examined, then followed for long periods to determine which arthritic diseases they developed and, if possible, what causative factors contributed to these diseases.

Plotting the distribution of different types of arthritis in worldwide population studies has yielded important clues to why the diseases occur. For example, the frequency of ankylosing spondylitis varies appreciably; it is common among the Haida Indians in the Queen Charlotte Islands off the coast of British Columbia, but it is uncommon in Japan. Post-dysenteric reactive arthritis appears to be more common in Nordic countries; it is suspected that this may be due to a genetic factor. In Papua, New Guinea, there is a markedly increased frequency of what is believed to be reactive arthritis, for which there is no adequate explanation. Different frequencies of psoriatic arthritis have been reported in various countries, possibly because of variation in the diagnostic criteria used. The frequency of rheumatoid arthritis is remarkably constant at 1 percent in almost all countries, except that it is less common in the African bush, in Polynesia, and in Puerto Rico.

In Chapter 7 I mentioned a proposal that rheumatoid arthritis may have been rare before 1800. There is now complementary evidence, from a 1980 study in Minnesota, that rheumatoid arthritis in women may be becoming less frequent. This thesis is debatable and has been denied by some experts. Yet recent reports from England, Seattle, and Finland all point in the same direction. If the evidence is to be believed, it raises questions about what causative factors were introduced in the past two hundred years that might have caused arthritis, and apparently are now declining.

From the first epidemiological studies of arthritis, one of the prime objectives has been to determine the importance of heredity and environment in causation. As we found with familial Mediterranean fever, cystic fibrosis, hemophilia, and gout, epidemiological investigations are comparatively simple when there is one gene and one disease, and the condition conveniently follows Mendel's laws. But most arthritis does not behave in this way, either clinically or genetically.

Until recently, when analyzing diseases such as ankylosing spondylitis, reactive arthritis, psoriatic arthritis, and rheumatoid arthritis, we depended mainly on studies of families, twins, populations, and races. Research on identical twins has been particularly valuable because when studying humans we cannot follow Mendel's example of selecting special varieties of seeds that create individual characteristics, or the geneticists' method of breeding pure strains of animals. Instead, we observe identical twins because we can follow what happens to people born with precisely the same genetic makeup. We can also compare them with nonidentical twins, who are born at the same time and have environments that are as alike as those shared by identical twins.

In ankylosing spondylitis, evidence of a hereditary factor was noted in families at an early stage of the investigation of the disease. Kellgren and his colleagues in 1968 published a family study in which clinical ankylosing spondylitis was present in 4 percent of close relatives of individuals with the disease, compared with 0.1 to 0.2 percent of the general population. This significant finding indicates a powerful genetic component—but it does not conform to Mendelian genetics.

Sexually acquired reactive arthritis is difficult to investigate. Nevertheless, in a family study published by Lawrence in 1974, there was a striking increase in the frequency of both psoriasis and ankylosing spondylitis in close relatives. This suggests the possibility that genes for both diseases may play a part in reactive arthritis.

Many researchers have investigated the family clustering of psoriasis and its associated arthritis. For instance, in 1973 Verna Wright and his colleagues at Leeds reported an investigation of families of people with psoriatic arthritis. In addition to the expected strong hereditary influence for psoriasis and arthritis, the genetic components separated out in the relatives, so that they had psoriasis, or peripheral arthritis, or spondylitis; but few relatives had psoriatic arthritis similar to the disease in the key member of the family.

Attempts to establish evidence of a hereditary element in rheumatoid arthritis have proved to be particularly difficult. By 1966, after several family and population studies of rheumatoid arthritis, the experts were unable to agree on whether the disease has a genetic component. Some researchers who had been involved in these studies decided that heredity had no role in causation. Kellgren concluded, "If a genetic predisposition to rheumatoid arthritis can be established, it is clearly very slight."

Stronger evidence for a hereditary component in rheumatoid arthritis has come from twin studies. When one identical twin has rheumatoid arthritis, the chance that the other twin will also develop the disease varies between 12 percent and 34 percent; the figure depends mainly on how the twins were identified in the community and included in the investigation. Comparable figures for nonidentical twins have varied between 4 percent and 10 percent. Because most twins with identical genes do not develop rheumatoid arthritis, the interpretation of these results is that other influences are definitely more important in causation than genetic factors. Recent investigations of families in which two or more close relatives have rheumatoid arthritis (implying a strong genetic influence) show a distinct increase of thyroid disease in these families.

The epidemiological evidence relating to factors in the environment is impressive but still incomplete. Worldwide surveys of rheumatoid arthritis have failed to show differences that match the immense variation in the prevailing social conditions and in the prevailing infectious organisms. It is still a tragic fact that in some parts of the world half of the population is dead by the age of fifteen years. As we know, some countries continue to be plagued by infectious diseases that are no longer seen in more fortunate populations. Yet it seems that whatever the conditions, they do not materially alter the incidence of rheumatoid arthritis.

After reviewing the evidence, Kellgren suggested in 1966 that the findings of surveys on rheumatoid arthritis implied that there was either a single environmental factor operating equally throughout the world or a multiplicity of factors operating to varying degrees in different populations. Since then, international collaboration in epidemiological studies has made it highly unlikely that the answer to rheumatoid arthritis will be found in a single ubiquitous environmental factor.

No environmental factors are known to cause psoriatic arthritis, apart from an occasional link to injury or infection. Preliminary evidence relating to infections in the causation of ankylosing spondylitis is still controversial.

We have already recognized that sometimes it is hard to detect infection as the cause of arthritis in one individual. But epidemiological surveys have usually demonstrated connections between infection and arthritis in large groups of people, even when the organisms were dead. For example, Ilmari Paronen found it easy to relate 344 cases of reactive arthritis to 150,000 people with dysentery.

In the United States, parallels have been drawn between Lyme arthritis and rheumatoid arthritis, but in terms of epidemiology they are certainly not the same. In Lyme, Polly Murray observed a clustering of patients in a small area near some woods. Noting a seasonal incidence and the presence of ticks, she quickly recognized that she was witnessing an epidemic of arthritis due to an infectious agent. The same is not true, however, of our key diseases—ankylosing spondylitis, psoriatic arthritis, and rheumatoid arthritis. We have been seeking infectious agents in them for a hundred years without finding any.

It is difficult to conduct an epidemiological survey in Minnesota or Lancashire; to do so in rural areas of central Africa seems impossible. The practical problems are immense. Yet excellent reports have emerged, and we follow what happens in Africa with great interest. In Nigeria, rheumatoid arthritis is uncommon; it usually runs a benign course, and it often lacks rheumatoid factor. In 1968 Brian Greenwood (a British physician working in Nigeria) reported that all autoimmune diseases are rare in the region. Indeed, he made the interesting suggestion that endemic childhood infections with malaria and other parasites might generate resistance to autoimmune diseases in adult life. Although this may be so, other workers found that arthritis is rare among the Bantu in a region where they are not exposed to malaria.

Rheumatoid arthritis is rare throughout central Africa, even allowing for the lower average age of the population. Instead, an arthritis resembling reactive arthritis is seen more frequently than rheumatoid arthritis. Two studies by the same team of workers in southern Africa yielded other results of fundamental importance (which have since been confirmed by several reports from elsewhere in Africa). In blacks living in the bush, rheumatoid arthritis was rare and mild; but in similar black populations in urban areas, the same disease, assessed by the same people, was much worse and ten times as common. The arthritis was so severe that many patients died of the disease within three years; special clinics had to be opened for black people living in urban areas. An explanation of these striking observations may lie in the differences between the environments in rural and urban Africa, including infection, stress, air pollution, water supply, and diet. It appears that powerful causative factors in the environment are waiting to be identified. If it were possible to establish what they are and to remove them by preventive measures, it might be feasible to make arthritis less severe and less prevalent, not only in Africa but throughout the world—obviously an attractive goal with immense implications.

The identification of rheumatoid factor in the blood proved from the beginning to be unreliable as a guide to the frequency of clinical rheumatoid arthritis in populations. Nonetheless, rheumatoid factor has produced provocative results in different ways.

The Mini–Finland Health Survey is based on a prospective review of more than seven thousand people over the age of thirty years. They are from diverse parts of the country and were selected to enable comparisons of social aspects of disease. At the beginning of the study, details of the individuals were recorded and blood samples were stored for later analysis. The results have not yet been published, but so far several people in the survey have developed rheumatoid arthritis. More than four years before the arthritis began, few of these people had rheumatoid factor in their blood, whereas within four years of the onset of disease half of them did. There are three principal implications of these results: first, a biological process may be under way years before the onset of symptoms; second, when at last means of prevention are established, we will have a further guide to the people at risk; third, we need to rethink all the evidence concerning the presence of rheumatoid factor in populations.

Air pollution poses significant questions. In an early investigation Kellgren and Lawrence found that rheumatoid factor levels were highest in British populations subjected to air pollution caused by smoke. It is unfortunate that these studies have not been repeated. We do have extensive evidence that regular occupational exposure to silica or asbestos frequently leads to autoantibodies and rheumatoid factor in the blood. This finding is particularly interesting because silica has toxic effects on cells of the immune system and is damaging to macrophages.

People who smoke cigarettes were shown to have increased autoantibodies and rheumatoid factor when a large population was surveyed in Busselton, Australia. The same was true in Finland, where investigators confirmed increased levels of rheumatoid factor in smokers.

Apart from these limited findings on rheumatoid factor, we have no firm evidence that arthritis itself is related to air pollution. Nevertheless, smokers appear to develop rheumatoid arthritis more frequently, and smokers with established rheumatoid arthritis are more likely to have increased complications in the small blood vessels of their skin. The existing evidence may be debatable, but the implications are considerable.

Studies of occupational hazards provide convincing evidence of the importance of exposure to silica in the local atmosphere. In a long-term investigation of 1,021 male granite workers in Finland, classic rheumatoid arthritis with rheumatoid factor was found to be significantly increased. The average interval between the first exposure to silica and the onset of joint symptoms was as much as twenty-five years, and the likelihood of developing arthritis was related to the amount of exposure to silica.

Taken together, the epidemiological evidence on rheumatoid factor and on clinical arthritis suggests that substances inhaled by the lungs may be significant causative factors in arthritis and may have a cumulative effect over a long period. Although this evidence relates primarily to rheumatoid arthritis (because, being common, it is easier to investigate), one cannot help suspecting that these substances are also important in other types of arthritis. Remember that systemic sclerosis is undoubtedly related to several occupational hazards—including the inhalation of silica.

To my knowledge, the effect of water supply on common types of arthritis has not been investigated, despite the fact that there are theoretical reasons to believe that it might be relevant. Rheumatologists want to learn more about the presence in the water supply of live bacteria that do not result in clinical evidence of infection, and about the presence of the products of dead bacteria. Either could affect the onset or severity of arthritis.

The role of diet in arthritis remains uncertain. Despite the immense variation in the diets of people throughout the world, rheumatoid arthritis is remarkably evenly spread almost everywhere. Apart from specific conditions such as gout and Kashin-Beck disease, we have no epidemiological evidence that diet influences arthritis in any group of people.

There is no doubt that small quantities of proteins enter the bloodstream from the gut intestines, and one would expect them also to enter the joints. A few people suffer joint symptoms as a result of food allergy. So far we have only limited evidence for deciding whether such mechanisms are important in rheumatoid arthritis, ankylosing spondylitis, or psoriatic arthritis. The most persuasive study is a trial conducted in Oslo and published in 1991. Twenty-seven patients with established rheumatoid arthritis were put on a vegetarian diet for one year; twenty-six matched patients acted as controls. The patients on the vegetarian diet improved in all of the many measurements made, and that improvement lasted throughout the year. These results are as satisfactory as those in any trial of drugs for the treatment of rheumatoid arthritis; but they deserve a word of caution, for the diet in the trial was supervised by professionals and catered for the needs of each individual. If a vegetarian diet simply became the latest fad adopted by people treating their own arthritis, some of the consequences might be tragic.

At least two relevant results in animals have been reported. "Old English" rabbits fed on cows' milk developed an arthritis resembling rheumatoid arthritis; and pigs fed on a diet of fish meal underwent a proliferation of a particular type of bacteria in the intestines, followed by acute arthritis in many joints.

We have every reason to be grateful to Kellgren, Lawrence, and all the others who built up effective international collaboration and a large number of excellent academic departments devoted to the epidemiology of arthritis. My own opinion is that it would be impossible to invest too many resources in this approach. Epidemiology has already provided a bank of knowledge that will be the foundation of all future progress in understanding arthritis.

17

Self and Nonself

The next step, which has had remarkable consequences, depended on making a connection between two branches of science that seemed to be poles apart: the inherited susceptibility to arthritis and the rejection of skin grafts and organ transplants. To understand arthritis, it is now essential to learn in detail how the body recognizes foreign substances and how we inherit the capacity to achieve this remarkable recognition.

Fortunately for all of us, throughout this century a whole science has built up around blood transfusion, skin grafting, and organ transplantation. Although the research was not done with arthritis in mind, since 1971 this new subject has transformed our approach to arthritis and has assisted the search for its causes more than any other development in the history of medicine. Yet the subject is complicated and technical. As with arthritis, distinct lines of research and discovery from different directions have contributed to our knowledge of transfusion and transplantation, so a simple account is impossible.

Undaunted, I start with blood transfusion. In 1657 the architect Sir Christopher Wren was the first to demonstrate the value of rehydration by injecting fluid into veins. During the next few years, many experiments followed in which animals were given blood transfusions. But it was not until 1829 that James Blundell, an obstetrician at Guy's Hospital in London, successfully gave a blood transfusion to a woman with excessive bleeding at delivery.

Blood transfusion must have been an extremely hazardous process throughout the nineteenth century; it had never been investigated.

Scientists had worked on immunity to bacteria and bacterial toxins, but only at the end of the century did they take up reactions to transfusion. It was Jules Bordet (1870–1961), a superb investigator at the Pasteur Institute, who first put transfusion on a scientific basis. He followed up experiments by Paul Ehrlich and showed in 1898 that when rabbits' blood is injected into guinea pigs, it produces a protective substance in the guinea pigs' serum that can destroy rabbit red blood cells. Two years later, Ehrlich proved that this principle did not depend on using two different species but applied also to serum from the same species. He demonstrated that rabbit serum could be made to destroy rabbit red blood cells.

In 1900 Karl Landsteiner (1868–1943), then an assistant in the Department of Pathological Anatomy in Vienna, discovered the ABO blood groups of human red blood cells. He showed that when a person is given a transfusion of blood from another person, the red blood cells may clump and be destroyed. Transfusions had been used for decades: Landsteiner proposed that this clumping explained the shock and jaundice that had occurred after mismatched blood transfusions for so many years. Later the ABO blood groups were found to be inherited. At that point two types of red blood cell, A and B, were known; and the genes for those two characteristics were dominant. So the inheritance of ABO groups follows Mendel's laws: you can have A, or B, or both (AB), or neither (O)—like Mendel's seeds. Landsteiner went on to show that a transfusion of B type to a person with B group, or a transfusion of A type to a person with A group, caused no reaction. Catastrophe occurred only when blood was given to someone with a different group, raising the all-important question of how the body knew that the wrong blood was foreign.

During World War I conditions in Vienna deteriorated, and by 1919 the medical facilities were so bad that Landsteiner felt obliged to move to the Netherlands for three years, before going on to the Rockefeller Institute for Medical Research in New York. Although he did not participate, much work on transplantation was being conducted there. Perhaps because of this association, in 1930 Landsteiner suggested that tissue cells might contain a system similar to blood groups, which would govern the acceptance or rejection of tissue transplants just as blood groups determine transfusion reactions. In subsequent years, particularly during World War II, many people added other blood groups. Landsteiner was among them, and he collaborated in discovering rhesus blood groups in 1940.

*   *   *

In looking at skin grafts and organ transplants, we turn the clock back four centuries. Gaspare Tagliacozzi of Bologna, who could be regarded as the father of plastic surgery, must have been a remarkable man. In "De Curtorum Chirurgia per Insitionem," written in 1597, he described operations in which he had replaced a mutilated nose—two hundred fifty years before the introduction of anesthesia. He detached one end of a flap of skin from the forearm and attached it to the face, at first leaving the other end joined to the forearm so that it had a blood supply. Then, a few weeks later, he detached the graft from its original site in the fore-arm and completed the surgery of the face. With extraordinary insight (or unfortunate experience) Tagliacozzi knew that a graft could be taken from the individual but not from another person. He attributed this re-jection of someone else's tissues to the "force and power" of the individ-ual. Sadly, until the early nineteenth century, his pioneering work—like that of Mendel and many others—was forgotten.

The next step in the history of transplantation came in 1869, when a young house surgeon, Jacques Louis Reverdin, recognized that in mak-ing skin grafts it is advisable to prepare thin grafts into which new blood vessels from the recipient's tissues can grow quickly. Reverdin intro-duced *lambeaux cutanes*—thin, minute grafts that are still used exten-sively, not only in surgery but also in the scientific investigation of trans-plantation. Despite such advances, a long, disastrous period followed in which surgeons ignored Tagliacozzi's advice and attempted to transplant skin and pieces of organs from one person to another, with dire results. They gradually learned the hard way that self soon recognizes nonself and destroys it.

At the start of this century a Danish scientist, C. O. Jensen, was the first to suggest that the rejection of a graft from one person by another person was a function of the immune system. Then it was the turn of a young surgeon named Alexis Carrel to make a major technical contri-bution to transplantation: Carrel (1873–1944), who was born in France and emigrated to Chicago, developed a technique for joining blood ves-sels end to end so that organs could be transplanted and given an im-mediate blood supply. When he moved to the Rockefeller Institute in 1906, he introduced a technique for perfusing the heart to keep it alive outside the body.

An indication of how much had been learned can be found in a book on transplantation published in 1912 and written by George Schone: it includes almost five hundred references. By this time many things were clear. For instance, it was known that a first graft from a different person is rejected after a delay, whereas a second graft is rejected almost immediately. It had also been established that in a graft between family members, the closer the relationship of the donor to the patient, the greater the likelihood of success—indicating a possible genetic component in graft rejection.

After a long pause when little changed in the clinical application of transplantation, the first kidney transplant took place in Kiev in 1933; unfortunately, the patient died two days later. A further delay of two decades followed before kidney transplants were successful—in Paris and Boston. In 1953 Joseph Murray, a surgeon at Brigham and Women's Hospital in Boston, carried out the first successful kidney transplant between identical twins. In the meantime, World War II had had a profound effect on the science of tissue transplantation, particularly skin grafts, just as it accelerated our knowledge of blood transfusion. Regular transplants of hearts, bone marrow, lungs, and other tissues and organs followed, bringing with them techniques and research of bewildering complexity.

Despite the advances and brilliant results during the first four decades of this century, it was a strange, rather confused period when experiments on the transplantation of normal tissues and of tumor tissues continued in parallel. A sense of this confusion can be gained from the experience of Peyton Rous (1879–1969), who joined the Rockefeller Institute in 1909 to concentrate on cancer research and to found the cancer research laboratory there. One of Rous's first projects was to study the differences in the body's reaction to grafts of normal tissue and grafts of tumor tissue. As he explained: "Much is now known of the behavior of transplantable tumors in the new host, of the conditions that regulate transplantation, and of the phenomena immediately concerned in growth or death of the introduced neoplasm (tumor); but there have been few attempts to determine what is here peculiar to tumor, as apart from transplanted tissues in general."

Almost as a side issue, while doing this research Rous discovered the first example of a virus that caused a malignant tumor—the Rous sarcoma virus in fowl. For this, he won the Nobel Prize.

James Murphy joined Rous in 1911 and decided to study not the acceptance of grafts but the factors that produced resistance to grafts. Soon, finding that lymphocytes play a key role in responses to grafts, Murphy began a systematic study of how cells affect graft rejection.

Apart from Rous, everyone was delighted with Murphy's work on lymphocytes. The Director of the Institute, the now-famous Simon Flexner, wrote, "It is needless to say that these results have a fundamental bearing on the problem of transplantation." Carrel, being a flamboyant surgeon, expressed his enthusiasm differently: "from a surgical standpoint the problem of graft rejection can be considered as having been solved." After these accolades, Murphy's advocacy of lymphocytes was forgotten for thirty years.

The investigation of responses in small animals to transplants of normal tissue and of tumor tissue continued unabated, now largely as a form of basic science. A key person in this work was a young American geneticist, Clarence C. Little. In 1914 he proposed a concept to explain how patients (or animals) could accept grafts from near relatives. His suggestion, later confirmed, was that donor and recipient must share important genes. Soon after, Little became President of the University of Maine. Although too busy to do research himself, he used his influence to help found the Jackson Memorial Laboratory in Bar Harbor, Maine. This institution took the lead in putting this type of genetics on a firm footing; it started by overcoming a difficult problem. Much as Mendel had studied seeds, animal geneticists studied mice because of the ease of conducting breeding experiments. At first the practice was unsatisfactory because individual mice had genes that were as dissimilar as those in individual humans. This period was later described as one of using "any old mice." An essential step was the development of strains of mice that were purebred and had virtually identical genes. These strains were then made available to laboratories everywhere, thereby radically altering experimental genetics throughout the world.

Peter (later Sir Peter) Gorer, working at Guy's Hospital in 1938, was the first to show that in purebred mice the rejection system was controlled by a certain set of genes. His investigation was extended by George Snell, a founder of transplantation genetics, who had worked at Bar Harbor since 1935 and later collaborated with Gorer. Subsequently, it was established that the genes for transplant rejection in the mouse are on the seventeenth chromosome.

Thus, we know that our bodies can recognize other people's blood, tissues, and organs, and that this ability is conveyed in our genes. Each of us inherits a system that characterizes us as an individual. Our ability to reject grafts separates us even from our families, so our body does not readily accept grafts from our closest relatives. The system for rejecting grafts is clearly far more sophisticated than the system for rejecting ABO blood groups.

We now need to consider together two men, an Australian and an Englishman, working a world apart: Macfarlane Burnet (1899–1985) and Peter Medawar (1915–1987), both of them later knighted. Although of different ages and working separately on different topics, much of what they did was complementary. In 1960 they shared the Nobel Prize "for their discovery of acquired immunological tolerance."

Peter Medawar, a brilliant young scientist working in Oxford, made a dramatic entry into the field of transplantation research during World War II. As he sat with his family in the garden, a lone British bomber crashed two hundred yards away. A young airman survived and was admitted to the Radcliffe Infirmary with severe burns. Although Medawar was not medically qualified, a colleague invited him to the bedside and asked if he could help with the difficult problem of skin grafting. The subject was new to Medawar, but the shock of being faced with this practical problem in such a forceful way resulted in his spending the rest of his life studying graft rejection. His dynamic personality stimulated many others to recognize the importance of the subject. In his approach to science, we see two features that he shared with Pasteur and other outstanding persons we have discussed: he had the capacity to recognize the basic mechanism underlying a problem, and he was unusually articulate.

Medawar's first action was to win support from the Medical Research Council to work at the Glasgow Royal Infirmary with an experienced plastic surgeon, Thomas Gibson. The two men quickly confirmed that a first graft from another individual is invaded by lymphocytes and rejected, whereas a graft from the patient is accepted. They also confirmed that, after a delay of a few days, the cells of the immune system recognize that the graft is foreign and react to destroy it. As a surgeon, Gibson already knew that a second foreign graft would not survive as long. He and Medawar showed that second grafts are destroyed immediately (reminiscent of Koch's discovery that an injection of dead tubercle bacilli will produce a severe reaction in an animal that has had a previous infection with tubercle bacilli). It is as though the immune cells have been warned.

After moving back to Oxford, Medawar conducted a classic series of experiments on small animals. He confirmed that the response to a first graft is not always present and occurs only after a latent period, whereas the response to a second graft is immediate. He also established that this accelerated response is specific to the original donor animal: grafts from different but similar animals are rejected more slowly.

You will remember that antibodies dominated immunology for the first four decades of this century. It is probably for this reason that Murphy's views on lymphocytes in transplantation were ignored, despite his prestigious position. By contrast, Medawar, even after his brief experience, was utterly convinced that the rejection of person-to-person grafts was dependent on cells, and he would not be dissuaded. When faced with the objection that "if there are no antibodies, it cannot be an immune response," he rightly commented, "Antibody formation is a tyrannical concept, and the hunt for antibodies has caused us to neglect other important strategies of defence."

Macfarlane Burnet, a virologist and microbiologist who had spent much of his career studying antibodies, wrote a monograph in 1941 stressing the role of cells in immune responses. Like Ehrlich and many after him, Burnet emphasized the problem involved in the body's recognizing and rejecting foreign substances while tolerating one's own tissues. In Burnet's opinion, the ability of the immune system to recognize and protect self is critical. Knowing that the mechanism for recognizing nonself is inherited and fully developed in the first cell of an embryo, and that full immunity is achieved more slowly, he proposed that the ability to tolerate self is learned early in embryonic life. He believed that the immune system stores a memory of self so that it can tolerate self throughout a person's life.

Medawar tested Burnet's hypothesis in mouse embryos and confirmed that immunological tolerance could be acquired. Within defined limits, the immune system could be taught to accept skin grafts from another animal, an observation that was very encouraging to surgeons investigating the use of grafts. A new world of immunology had been discovered.

The scene was set for a breakthrough that would have delighted Landsteiner. Jean Dausset, after a busy war, went to work in the basement of the Regional Blood Transfusion Center of the St.-Antoine Hospital in Paris. Because he was responsible for exchange transfusions in young

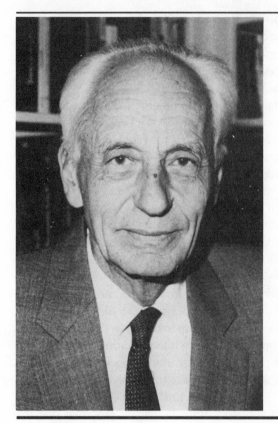

Jean Dausset, Nobel Laureate. Known as the father of HLA, Dausset discovered the HLA system, one of the great advances in the history of biological and medical science.

women following clandestine abortions, he was involved with antibodies against the patients' own red blood cells. His dream became antibodies against white blood cells, instead of against red cells, and he began to look for them.

One day in 1948 Dausset mixed fresh live white cells from one patient with the serum of a patient who had had many blood transfusions. To his astonishment, the white blood cells formed massive clumps, leaving no doubt that the serum contained a substance that had a powerful effect on white blood cells. Later he proved that a similar effect could be found in the serum of other people who had had multiple blood transfusions. The factor he found did not damage the person to whom it belonged—only the white blood cells of other people.

This situation was one such as Landsteiner had envisaged, but how was he to sort out the antibodies against white blood cells when the serum had been stimulated by many transfusions and presumably contained a complicated mixture of substances harmful to white cells? No computers were available to help, but Dausset was assisted by many researchers, including a delightful genius, the geneticist Ruggero Ceppellini, who had previously made the very important discovery of gene interaction. Among Ceppellini's suggestions was the use of a battery of white cell antibodies against the cells of identical and nonidentical twins—an invaluable approach.

After years of complicated work, in 1958 the first well-defined white cell antigen was born as the result of weekly injections of the same blood into volunteers (without knowing the genetic differences between them). From that exciting beginning came the routine testing of white cell types, called tissue-typing. Just as cross-matching of red blood cells is performed before blood transfusion, tissue-typing is now performed before organ transplantation. Just as Landsteiner's red cell groups were called ABO, Dausset's antigens became HLA antigens, from Human, Leukocyte (white cell), and A (the first antigen discovered).

After Dausset's pioneer work, scientists around the world soon joined in, including Amos, Bodmer, Ceppellini, Kissmeyer-Nielsen, Payne, Terasaki, van Rood, and Walford. In 1958 Jon van Rood (in Leiden) and Rose Payne (in Stanford) showed independently that antibodies are formed in pregnant women as a reaction to the fetus, which of course is foreign to the mother. For purposes of tissue-typing, finding antibodies in the serum of women with children had the immense advantage that this serum was readily available and far more specific than serum containing antibodies as the result of many transfusions.

Computers were soon busy, and international cooperation was seen at its very best. Competitiveness between scientists can act either as a powerful stimulus or as a major barrier to progress. Therefore, it has been heartwarming that everyone in the world involved in studying HLA antigens consented to collaborate wholeheartedly. From then on they agreed on international research programs, they met regularly, they pooled their results, and they published their findings jointly.

In 1964 a gifted scientist in Los Angeles, Paul Terasaki, reported (with John McClelland) a standard technique for tissue-typing that used small quantities of cells and serum under the microscope. Their technique was readily adopted as an international standard.

A seminal event in unraveling the HLA system and in putting tissue-typing on a sound footing was the Torino Workshop of 1967. Ruggero Ceppellini arranged for a group of Italian families to give blood daily for the workshop teams to analyze. This program enabled immense strides to be made in classifying HLA antigens. Looking back, many scientists appreciate how rare and precious were those moments at Torino; Ceppellini deserves much of the credit for what was achieved.

The next step was by Baruj Benacerraf and Hugh McDevitt, who discovered genes that determined specific immune responses in small animals. Years later, these proved to be the animal equivalent of a second extremely important class of HLA antigens in humans. Then the genes for the HLA antigens were found to be controlled by a mechanism on the sixth human chromosome.

Before long it was apparent that the whole subject had grown into something far larger than organ transplantation. Instead of four ABO groups, each human being has more than twenty-five HLA antigens (or molecules), all of which have many variations. Thus, millions of combinations of HLA molecules characterize us as individuals.

The HLA system is the principal mechanism by which our bodies tell the difference between self and nonself, and, as Burnet had said, that is a central function of the immune system. HLA has been essential in our evolution; it remains essential to human life. The discovery of this incredible system constitutes an advance in biological and medical science comparable in significance to the establishment of the germ theory of disease.

Forty years ago, to the surprise of many people, it was shown that there are weak links between some diseases and the red blood cell groups we inherit. Much later, the same approach was gradually applied to HLA and disease. In 1964 Frank Lilly of the Albert Einstein College of Medicine in the Bronx (New York) showed that mice with certain inherited molecules responded unusually to a virus infection. Three years later J. L. Amiel of the Hôpital Paul-Brousse in Villejuif reported a possible weak association in humans between an individual HLA molecule and Hodgkin's disease, a finding that has never been satisfactorily confirmed. At the same meeting Dausset reported a study of leukemia that showed no association.

During the next few years no persuasive results emerged. In retrospect, many of the diseases investigated then were the ones familiar to the researchers working with HLA, rather than the most suitable diseases. It is a measure of the specialization in modern medicine that most of us in other fields had no idea that these studies were under way. Meaningful links between HLA and disease were not established until five years or more after Amiel's initial paper. Nevertheless, it was always only a matter of time before they would be found.

As with the search for bacteria, many of the contributions to understanding blood transfusion and organ transplantation have been recognized officially. Of the scientists mentioned in this chapter Bordet, Ehrlich, and Rous were awarded the Nobel Prize for other work. Landsteiner, Carrel, Burnet, Medawar, Snell, Benacerraf, Dausset, and Murray won Nobel Prizes for contributions to blood transfusion, transplantation, or inherited mechanisms that distinguish self from nonself. There is widespread agreement that Gorer would have won a Nobel Prize if he had lived. The whole subject has seen such a dramatic advance that I am not alone in wishing that others too had become Nobel laureates.

18

The Race for Answers

It is always difficult to retain at the top of the agenda the problems that have no accepted answers. Although most rheumatologists by now have forgotten, until the 1970s they found it hard to keep before them the evidence that there is a hereditary component in arthritis. The results from studies of families, twins, and races were persuasive, but few of the findings fitted readily into a simple Mendelian pattern as did cystic fibrosis and hemophilia. Above all, no mechanism explained how one could inherit a tendency to inflammation. Most of us thought that these observations were important—and then set them aside.

My own opportunity to make a contribution to this story came when I least expected it. On a glorious English summer day in 1971, I had just completed a long and difficult clinic devoted to people with arthritis. Arriving late for lunch in the consultants' dining room at Westminster Hospital, I happened to sit at a table with my colleague David James, the head of our tissue-typing laboratory. He had just returned from an international meeting of transplantation immunologists, where they had discussed again the possible relation between HLA and disease. David had spare laboratory space and facilities, and he was asking fellow consultants in many specialties whether they could propose suitable diseases to study. To my surprise, no one had any suggestions.

I thought about this over my salad. Most of my patients had unexplained inflammation of their joints; in many of them, their arthritis had a hereditary component. Ankylosing spondylitis was the best example. Still, HLA molecules were inherited and connected to immune response genes. Over the coffee, I asked David if we could tissue-type a series of

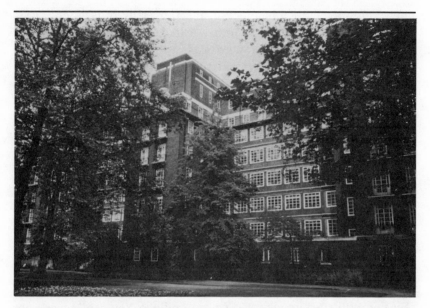

Westminster Hospital. First established in 1720, the hospital is currently situated near Westminster Abbey and the Houses of Parliament.

patients with ankylosing spondylitis. To me, ankylosing spondylitis was a disease bedeviled by attacks of inflammation—in the joints, in the eyes, and in the spine. Years later I learned to my surprise that scientists unfamiliar with this disease thought of it as simply a rigid condition of the spine, as indicated by its name. To immunologists it was a dull disease: after all, there were no antibodies. I do not know what Medawar might have said, but I was interested not so much in antibodies as in inflammation in people.

Anyway, after lunch David and I went to my office nearby, and I dug out all of the literature about family studies and population surveys of ankylosing spondylitis. We agreed to go ahead. I would assess the patients from a clinical point of view, and he would supervise the tissue-typing. After delays in obtaining financial support, we started on the project, thanks to a grant from the Board of Governors of Westminster Hospital.

I was joined by a new senior registrar (medical resident), Anne Nicholls, who was indispensable in organizing and carrying out much of the clinical work. At the beginning we were helped by Roger Sturrock, now Professor of Rheumatology at the University of Glasgow. David Walters, a postgraduate fellow from Australia, later became part of the team. David James recruited Maeve Caffrey to do the tissue-typing with the technique devised by Terasaki and McClelland. David and Maeve did all the laboratory work, and without their expertise the project would have been impossible. We were a happy and efficient team.

But there were immediate problems. One of my tasks was to remember as many as possible of the people with ankylosing spondylitis we had seen recently, because in those days we did not have a diagnostic index. (Ever since, we have kept cards indicating our main diagnoses of each patient, so it is easy to locate patients with particular diseases. But not then.) We also had to devise a system of assessing each patient. Like Mendel with his seeds, we had to record separately the different clinical characteristics in each patient, because HLA might be related to some clinical features but not others.

Moreover, we had to avoid bias. We agreed that Anne and I would record all the clinical details, and at a weekly meeting Maeve would present the results before we revealed our findings. You can imagine our astonishment and excitement when, at our first meeting, all eight patients with ankylosing spondylitis were found to have what was then a new HLA molecule, now known as HLA-B27, or B27 for short. This molecule is present in 8 percent of the British population, so the possibility of finding the same molecule in eight patients by chance is less than one in a million. The same afternoon, and again the following day, Anne and I met in my office to decide what to do next. I remember vividly my sense of awe at the responsibility that had fallen on my shoulders.

The first decisions were easy. We would need about a hundred patients with ankylosing spondylitis and would have to assess their clinical features, family histories, laboratory findings, and x-rays. As this was not a population survey and the accepted diagnostic criteria were not sufficiently strict, we would have to formulate our own criteria in order to exclude patients in whom there was any doubt of the diagnosis. At the same time, we planned several other projects that were to start immediately but would not be given priority or reported until later. (As it turned out, we knew the answers to the questions they posed before our first paper on ankylosing spondylitis was published.)

It was difficult to carry on this research and a full load of clinical work as well; but slowly and painstakingly, and with remarkable cooperation from our patients, the figures mounted: B27 in twenty-four of twenty-

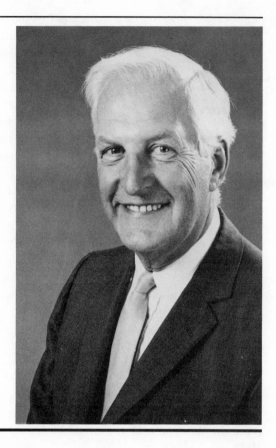

Derrick Brewerton.

five, then forty-eight of fifty. It seemed too good to be true. I worried whether it might be a false result, produced not in the laboratory but in the patients. Could radiotherapy or drugs have modified the results? Viewed in retrospect, these were mad ideas, but they caused me nightmares at the time. Then there was the more logical fear that some unknown feature of the disease might have influenced our results. For instance, could a persistent virus in the cells alter the HLA molecule?

I struck on a ready solution. HLA molecules, inherited according to Mendel's laws, are dominant and not sex linked. Most of the close (first-degree) relatives would not have the disease and would not have had any treatment. But if the HLA molecule was inherited normally, half of the relatives of patients with B27 should also have B27. We knew the family histories, and by then we knew the patients and many of their families. So, day after day, Anne and I would set out from our respective homes at five in the morning to visit families around London. In all manner of dwellings we drank tea after examining our hosts and taking blood samples before they went off to work. To my intense relief, we found that thirty-two of sixty relatives had B27, and it was correctly distributed between the sexes and among the different types of relatives. Of the twenty-nine adult relatives with B27, three had ankylosing spondylitis and seven more had symptoms suggestive of spondylitis. By contrast, only one of the relatives without B27 had backache.

Then we came to the vexing question of publication, to which I still do not know the answer. When, in 1972, I chaired a meeting in my office to discuss the matter, David James correctly advocated early publication to establish scientific priority. I was torn. I knew that the article we wrote would be much read and frequently quoted. I wanted to investigate enough patients to see if any clinical features occurred in the absence of B27; I wanted to finish the family studies; and I wanted to complete my literature review to provide an authoritative background to the article that it would be my responsibility to write. Rightly or wrongly, we decided to compromise.

By the time the article I wrote was finished, we had found B27 in seventy-two of seventy-five patients, three of seventy-five controls, and thirty-two of sixty relatives. This meant that someone born with HLA-B27 was three hundred times as likely as other individuals to develop ankylosing spondylitis later in life. Between us, we published a short report in *Nature* in March 1973 and a full account in the *Lancet* in April 1973.

I have already mentioned that Paul Terasaki of Los Angeles is a pioneer in the subject of HLA and kidney transplants and designed (with McClelland) the standard technique for tissue-typing. A leader in the study of associations between HLA and disease, he is now the undoubted world authority on the subject. After his technique was announced in 1964, Terasaki continued to improve it; he advanced to a stage where everything was automated and he could study the tissue types of all the patients admitted to his large hospital at UCLA. As he wrote to me recently, "We operated on the thesis that there was no way to predict which disease would be associated by any armchair guessing." In the long term, he has been right—many unanticipated associations have turned up.

Rodney Bluestone, an English rheumatologist who had emigrated to

Los Angeles a few years earlier, was invited to send blood samples to Terasaki for tissue-typing. With good reason, he decided to study gout. He wrote later:

The way the whole thing happened was rather remarkable. During 1972, I was interested in studying tissue-types of patients with typical gout. We wanted control groups, and one of the selected control groups was patients with ankylosing spondylitis, i.e., patients with another well-defined rheumatic disease, the majority of them male. The first 20 patients that we typed from this control group came back with a 95% incidence of HLA-B27, which was then a fairly newly recognized antigen . . . I must say that, at the time we stumbled across the remarkable correlation, Paul Terasaki was about the only person in town who really understood the significance of tissue-typings and their probable association to immune response genes.

The Los Angeles group then suffered delays, just as we had suffered delays. They had the frustration of having an article rejected. Consequently, their report in the *New England Journal of Medicine* of HLA-B27 in thirty-five of forty patients with ankylosing spondylitis was not published until April 1973—midway between the two Westminster articles. By then both groups had learned how easily scientific priority can be influenced by factors unrelated to scientific merit. Having a strong dislike of competitiveness in science, I regard the outcome as a dead heat between two groups who, unknown to each other, had worked long and hard on the same project. I stand by what I said in the Bunim Lecture to the American Rheumatism Association in 1975: "The discovery of the relationship between ankylosing spondylitis and HLA-B27 was made independently and simultaneously in Westminster and Los Angeles. The credit for this finding and the honour of this lecture should be shared by all of us in both groups."

Of course, Rodney Bluestone and I had checked that B27 is not associated with rheumatoid arthritis. We at Westminster had also shown that B27 is not found more frequently than normal in two disorders that are similar to ankylosing spondylitis, particularly in their x-ray appearances: vertebral hyperostosis and osteitis condensans ilii.

We now return to the research projects Anne Nicholls and I had planned at the outset. Although ankylosing spondylitis came first in our research at Westminster, by far our most important discovery related to the type of reactive arthritis described so long ago by Sir Benjamin Brodie. Despite the differences early in the disease, sexually acquired reactive arthritis closely resembles ankylosing spondylitis in its disorders of the spine, peripheral joints, and eyes. The research significance of the disease is that, unlike ankylosing spondylitis, it follows infection and therefore could reveal the mechanism that enables organisms to enter the joints undetected.

Men with sexually acquired reactive arthritis are often young and socially mobile; hence they are difficult to recall for investigation. With help from colleagues and the Army, we managed to examine enough young men: thirty-three controls, thirty-three with genital infection without joint disease, and thirty-three with sexually acquired reactive arthritis. B27 was present in two controls and in three men with genital infection, an indication that B27 does not predispose to the initial infection. The tissue-typing results for those with arthritis were crucial: B27 was present in twenty-five of the thirty-three men. This meant that men born with B27 who contract a genital infection are almost one hundred times more likely than those without B27 to suffer arthritis a few weeks later. We also found that although the association between B27 and early peripheral arthritis is strong, even stronger is the association between B27 and the subsequent development of spondylitis, sacroiliitis, or uveitis—which rarely occur in the absence of B27. At last the complicated clinical associations between various diseases were beginning to fit into place.

By then we knew that B27 does not influence the likelihood of the initial inflammation of the genital tract; instead, like the rejection of grafts and transplants, this HLA molecule has a powerful effect on the delayed response after a few weeks. Just as graft rejection is specific to the individual, the genes that determine which HLA molecules we inherit also determine whether we develop arthritis as a consequence of foreign organisms entering the body. This observation is fundamental to the present understanding of arthritis.

Our investigations of acute anterior uveitis were also invaluable. To a clinician familiar with spondylitis, uveitis does not behave like a complication of spondylitis but like a different disease in the same individual. Thinking about this strange situation, I concluded that the link between the two diseases might be genetic and that if we were fortunate, we might prove it. I sought the advice of Edward Perkins, then Professor of

Ophthalmology at the Institute of Ophthalmology in London. An international authority on uveitis and author of the best monograph on the subject (based on a study of nearly two thousand patients), Perkins was most helpful. He warned me that there was no evidence that acute anterior uveitis might be inherited, but promised that he and his colleagues would do everything possible to help. And they did. New patients with acute anterior uveitis were asked whether they wished to volunteer to see me. During the next ten years more than eight hundred people with uveitis consulted me; and, to their advantage, I diagnosed almost two hundred previously unsuspected cases of spondylitis.

Of the first hundred patients with uveitis whom I saw, thirty had either spondylitis or a closely related form of arthritis. All but one of these thirty patients had B27, but that did not answer my question because the B27 might have been related to the arthritis and not to the uveitis. That left seventy people with acute anterior uveitis and no evidence of other disease. In them, B27 was present in twenty-nine patients (compared with six controls) and was equally divided between the sexes. This meant that a young person in London with B27 was twenty times as likely to go to the eye hospital with this painful complaint as the rest of the population. Furthermore, we noted an interesting relation to age: the people with B27 had their first attack of uveitis ten years earlier than did those without B27.

We had established, for the first time, the principle that two different diseases could be linked to the same HLA gene. We also knew that ankylosing spondylitis and reactive arthritis are separate diseases because, at the least, the early clinical features are different, and ankylosing spondylitis is not caused by genital infection or aggravated by any other symptomatic infection—even if the late features of the two diseases are virtually the same. We could see that the relationship of these two diseases to B27 could account for some clinical features being the same in both. We had discovered something new: three distinct common diseases—spondylitis, reactive arthritis, and uveitis—strongly associated with one gene.

Next we tackled the extraordinary overlapping clinical associations between ulcerative colitis, Crohn's disease, psoriasis, ankylosing spondylitis, peripheral arthritis, and acute anterior uveitis. To physicians, this remarkable collection of diseases is almost as complicated as the heredity of HLA molecules. They constitute nine forms of chronic inflammation of unknown cause: two in the intestines, one in the skin, one in the spine, four in the peripheral joints, and one in the eyes. They occur separately or together; when together, they are found in almost any combination far more often than could happen by chance. For example, people with these skin or bowel diseases develop spondylitis about twenty-five times more often than does the rest of the population.

The critical clue is that ulcerative colitis, Crohn's disease, psoriasis, and ankylosing spondylitis run in families, with comparable evidence of a hereditary component in each. Thus, one possibility was that these diseases are linked by heredity, as spondylitis and uveitis are linked. Up to a point this is true, but the full story proved to be far more complicated than we expected.

Our first task was to adopt definitions of the individual clinical features of the diseases. We then mapped out the combinations of those features that we would need to investigate in order to untangle this interwoven skein of disorders. After that, we contacted many friends and colleagues in and around London, and took full advantage of the cooperative nature of the National Health Service. This part of our research is a superb example of enthusiastic collaboration among doctors and patients. Gastroenterologists, dermatologists, rheumatologists, ophthalmologists, radiologists, and orthopedic surgeons in more than twenty-five hospitals went to endless trouble in searching their records and contacting patients who fulfilled our criteria. Then patients either volunteered to travel to Westminster, or one of us visited them in their hospitals or at home to examine them and take blood for tests.

In ulcerative colitis and Crohn's disease alone or with peripheral arthritis, the distribution of HLA antigens was normal. But when these inflammatory bowel diseases were associated with ankylosing spondylitis, B27 was present in over 60 percent, compared with 8 percent of controls. Before then, clinicians had loosely thought of spondylitis as a complication of the bowel diseases—although they appreciated that this assumption did not fit the facts. From our research we had demonstrated that the bowel and spinal disorders are separate biological processes linked by heredity, which conformed neatly with the clinical evidence.

Psoriasis was similar but more complicated, because psoriasis itself has a weak association with two other HLA molecules. In psoriatic arthritis without spondylitis we discovered a further weak association with B27. When spondylitis is present, B27 is again found in over 60 percent of patients, with the frequency of B27 corresponding to the severity of the spinal disease. At that stage I began to think of psoriasis, peripheral arthritis, and spondylitis as three separate processes occurring in these individuals.

In more than a third of those with psoriasis and spondylitis, the gene for psoriasis came from one parent and the gene for spondylitis from the other parent. That is true multigenic heredity.

Next was the issue of those who developed ankylosing spondylitis without B27. When I reviewed the patients in our studies, I found that half of those who had spondylitis without B27 had either bowel or skin disease; I postulated that in the other half the genes for bowel and skin disease might substitute for B27 in an unknown way. Thus, a man without B27 and ulcerative colitis had a daughter without B27 or colitis who, nevertheless, developed typical ankylosing spondylitis. Also, the unfortunate individuals who had several clinical features, including spondylitis, often did not have B27. It was as if the presence of many genes for other disorders made B27 unnecessary.

I was also puzzled by the relations between HLA, psoriasis, and the distribution of the joints involved in arthritis. For example, when I reviewed all the patients with B27 and spondylitis and looked at which peripheral joints were affected, finger arthritis was rare. But when psoriasis was present in a patient or in his or her family, finger arthritis was present in the majority, suggesting that genes related to those for psoriasis might predispose to finger disease.

The reports on B27 from Westminster and Los Angeles were not the first positive associations with disease. In 1972 Terasaki and his collaborators had reported weak but significant associations between HLA and both psoriasis and multiple sclerosis. Yet B27 has remained the strongest and most interesting of the associations. One distinguished pioneer, Hugh McDevitt, has written that it "threw a cloak of scientific respectability over the whole field of HLA and disease associations."

Soon after our first publications I was approached by an old friend, Geraint James of the Royal Northern Hospital in London. He was looking after one thousand people with sarcoidosis and had stored the clinical details on computer. We decided to follow the now familiar technique of concentrating on one clinical feature at a time, investigating all of the patients who had only one or two outstanding clinical features. To our surprise, the groups of people with erythema nodosum, or acute arthritis, or both erythema nodosum and acute arthritis, had an increased frequency of HLA-B8. This meant that someone who inherited B8 and then had sarcoidosis was ten times more likely to develop erythema nodosum or arthritis. From there we could speculate. For instance, B8 is much less common in Japan than in England, and patients with sarcoidosis in Japan seldom have erythema nodosum. Perhaps HLA could explain the different distributions of some diseases in different countries.

Finally, as I reviewed these findings, I pondered Koch's view that there is a different organism for each disease, with heredity perhaps influencing the susceptibility to that disease. Could it be the other way around in some diseases? With this form of heredity—and taking into account age, gender, hormones, nerves, stress, emotions, nutrition, and other host factors—together they might determine the nature and distribution of the disease response, the details of the clinical features, and the time at which an individual is most susceptible. If that were true, then the role of foreign organisms and substances could be nonspecific. Any trigger might do.

Scientists in many other disciplines, fascinated by the associations between arthritis and HLA, immediately wanted to know more about arthritis. Researchers who had not previously taken an interest in joint diseases soon appreciated that the best models to study were the people with arthritic diseases. In their turn, the patients and their families were only too delighted to contribute by helping with research projects, often at great inconvenience to themselves. Almost overnight, the search for the causes of arthritis shot from being a Cinderella endeavor to being one of the burning medical topics of the day. This welcome scientific boom came just as many powerful new techniques were blossoming in biological research. Largely because of those developments, the whole approach to arthritis research was transformed. As one facet of this new era, many millions of dollars were spent all over the world investigating not only HLA but all aspects of the genetics of arthritis. For more than a decade we had an exciting period in which the tissue-typing of people with all kinds of diseases was a major industry and the subject of worldwide cooperation.

Nevertheless, until about 1987 we did not understand how inherited HLA molecules could render people susceptible to arthritis. At first we were not even certain whether a molecule such as B27 was a fundamental part of the arthritis or merely an interesting marker for a more important neighboring gene that was more directly involved in the disease process.

The first response to our initial publications brought me great pleasure. For a long time, an impressive group in Finland had been studying post-dysenteric arthritis. Indeed, this group had introduced the term "reactive arthritis." On reading our results in the *Lancet*, they tissue-typed patients with post-dysenteric reactive arthritis, including many in whom the causative bacteria had been positively identified. Like our results with sexually acquired reactive arthritis, they found that people with HLA-B27 who had infections with these organisms were one hundred times as likely as other individuals to develop arthritis a few weeks later. This was an important advance because it meant that everyone could investigate the relationship among HLA molecules, bacteria, and arthritis—a combination that has remained one of the most attractive models for research ever since.

Month by month we learned from the reports of B27 in different countries. The most significant finding was that the link between B27 and ankylosing spondylitis was present everywhere, even in the most remote parts of the world. The experts in population genetics told us this could happen only if B27 itself were directly involved in the disease, so the alternative possibility of a neighboring gene was ruled out. We then knew for certain that our two groups, in Westminster and Los Angeles, had discovered that an inherited molecule plays a critical role in several common types of arthritis.

Enough exceptions to this link between B27 and ankylosing spondylitis proved the rule. For instance, in Tunisia and among American black people the relation between B27 and ankylosing spondylitis was reduced, which raised again the question of how a disease linked to a single gene can occur, with all the sophisticated details of that disease, in the absence of the gene concerned. This is a question that requires an answer.

Looked at another way, the frequency of B27 in some countries accounted for the variation in the prevalence of ankylosing spondylitis. For example, B27 is present in 50 percent of the Haida Indians in British Columbia but in only 1 percent of the people of Japan, thus explaining the high and low prevalence of ankylosing spondylitis in those populations. Even in such extreme situations, however, the link between B27 and the disease is as strong as anywhere else. Recent studies in northeast

Russia and along the shores of Alaska have revealed a concentration of B27 and ankylosing spondylitis on both sides of the Bering Strait, possibly related to the early migration of American native peoples.

Worldwide, the frequency of rheumatic symptoms in people with B27 selected at random within the local population was surprisingly low at 1 percent, or at most less than 2 percent. So the next crucial question was how 98 percent of people with B27 could remain free of symptoms throughout their life. It cannot be because everywhere in the world these people are not exposed to relevant trigger factors. Other missing ingredients in the individuals themselves must make them either more or less resistant to ankylosing spondylitis.

Careful family studies, in the Netherlands and in the United States, have investigated the close relatives of people with B27 and ankylosing spondylitis. In people with B27 and ankylosing spondylitis in their families, the frequency of this disease is twenty times as great as in people with B27 in the population at large. The implication is that at least one other genetic component in these families has yet to be found, and that this missing component is almost certain to be closely linked to B27.

With help from molecular biologists, B27 has been split into seven subtypes, all of which seem to be equally associated with disease. Yet population studies indicate that the subtypes are so widespread in races throughout the world that they must have developed at a time close to the origins of man. Therefore, either the link between B27 and ankylosing spondylitis is extremely primitive or the involvement of B27 in the disease process is not what we imagine. Both alternatives are intriguing.

In the last chapter I mentioned a second class of HLA molecules—the human equivalents of immune response genes in animals. These class II molecules are difficult to investigate, or at least they were when they were being discovered. In 1973 facilities for testing class II molecules were not widely available, but these molecules were destined to become in many ways more important than class I, to which B27 belongs.

While many of us were shaking our heads about the assumed weakness of any hereditary component in rheumatoid arthritis and contemplating the complexities of the new HLA molecules, Peter Stastny of Dallas triumphed. In 1974, after much elaborate work, he reported results that led to the identification of a genetic component in rheumatoid arthritis. With the advantage of hindsight, we now know that his inge-

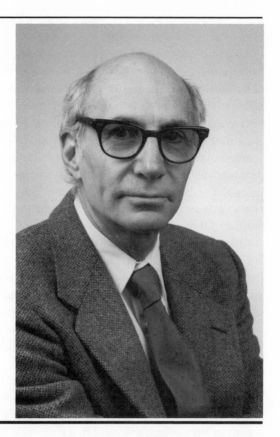

Peter Stastny. Now Professor of Internal Medicine at Southwestern Medical School in Dallas, Stastny uncovered the association between HLA molecules and rheumatoid arthritis.

nious technique indicated in an indirect way that just as there are different types of class I molecules, there also are different types of class II molecules.

At the same time, Robert Winchester, then working at Rockefeller University, defined class II molecules in human beings more clearly and more directly. This direct definition had not been achieved previously because it had been expected that class II molecules would be on all cells, as class I molecules are on all cells. Winchester's discovery depended on separating different types of cells and showing that class II molecules are normally found on B-cells and antigen-presenting cells, but not on T-cells. Stastny and Winchester independently used this new method to establish that people with HLA-DR4 are seven times as likely as others to develop rheumatoid arthritis—a figure that is in keeping with the epidemiological evidence that the influence of heredity in rheumatoid arthritis is not strong.

Although this excellent work was confirmed in most countries, surprises emerged. In Greeks, Israeli Jews, Bengalis, and Indians, the class II molecule associated with rheumatoid arthritis was not DR4 but another molecule, often DR1. For several years it appeared that DR4 and DR1 could not both be directly involved in rheumatoid arthritis in the way that B27 was in ankylosing spondylitis and other diseases. It seemed that the DR4 association that led to arthritis in northern Europe progressively lost its influence as one moved to southern Europe and crossed the Bosporus. This trend was perplexing because the class II types such as DR4 were widely thought to be the functional units that regulated the immune response.

Characteristic clear thinking guided Winchester's subsequent work. He recalled certain test sera that reacted highly specifically with blood from people with rheumatoid arthritis. He reasoned that the DR4 molecule, instead of being uniform, might differ slightly but significantly among ethnic groups. Winchester was joined by Peter Gregersen, who set about determining the molecular sequences of all genes related to DR4 in various ethnic groups. When the sequences were completed and assembled on the office desk, it was evident that DR4 molecules from ethnic groups whose DR4 was associated with rheumatoid arthritis differed from DR4 molecules in ethnic groups that had no such association.

The difference lay in several critical amino acids, all located in a small region of the molecule. Could this region be the site of susceptibility to rheumatoid arthritis? Winchester and Gregersen postulated correctly that the types of DR4 molecules that led to rheumatoid arthritis had specific features that were lacking in other varieties of DR4. The correctness of their notion was supported by establishing sequences of DR1 genes in patients with rheumatoid arthritis. Even though many widespread differences from DR4 were revealed, to everyone's fascination DR1 and DR4 molecules shared an identical genetic element when associated with rheumatoid arthritis. Further studies have confirmed that this tiny portion of the gene is likely to be the molecular basis of genetic susceptibility to rheumatoid arthritis.

At this point you will realize that certain HLA molecules are now believed to play a central role in our four most enigmatic types of arthritis: ankylosing spondylitis, reactive arthritis, psoriatic arthritis, and rheumatoid arthritis, as well as in psoriasis and acute anterior uveitis. That list alone indicates that HLA molecules are directly involved in the causation of disease in about 80 million people.

We have reached an appropriate juncture to reconsider the frequent marked improvement in the severity of rheumatoid arthritis during pregnancy. The many possible explanations for this phenomenon have centered on changes in the sex hormones—and some of these explanations may be correct.

Another suggestion is based on the conflict between self and nonself. After all, the embryo is foreign to the mother; it is one of the most remarkable facts in nature that the mother's immune system can tolerate in her bloodstream the steady input of foreign material from the fetus. Since it has been established that HLA molecules, so actively engaged in tolerance, are related to the basic processes of rheumatoid arthritis, one possibility has been that the improvement in the severity of disease is associated with the body's tolerance. Put simply, the mother's immune system may be so preoccupied with tolerating the embryo that it can no longer sustain active arthritis. This observation is supported by evidence that the arthritis improves only when there is a marked difference in the HLA molecules in the mother and the father, and therefore the mother and the embryo, so that the threat to tolerance is greater.

In reviewing the associations between HLA molecules and other types of arthritis mentioned in this book, we see how prominent a role HLA plays.

- The different types of arthritis in childhood, and the insidious uveitis in childhood, are associated with HLA molecules.
- Lyme disease, sarcoid erythema nodosum, "AIDS arthritis," polymyalgia rheumatica, Behçet's disease, and systemic sclerosis are all believed to have some form of association with HLA molecules. In Lyme disease, for example, Steere and Winchester showed that people with certain HLA molecules are more likely than other individuals to be troubled by the severity of some clinical features of their condition.
- Certain clinical aspects of common arthritic diseases have HLA links of their own—for example, the scarring of the lungs (fibrosing alveolitis) and the dry eyes and mouth (Sjögren's syndrome) sometimes encountered in rheumatoid arthritis. We even have evidence that the

way we respond to certain drugs used in the treatment of arthritis is linked to HLA.

By contrast, diseases like familial Mediterranean fever, cystic fibrosis, hemophilia, and gout—which follow Mendel's laws and probably have comparatively simple genetic links—are not included in the list of diseases associated with HLA.

Many organ-specific autoimmune diseases have proved to be associated with HLA molecules. These include juvenile diabetes, thyrotoxicosis, thyroiditis, and myasthenia gravis. And some features of SLE are associated with HLA molecules.

Several important diseases *not* clinically linked to arthritis have associations with the HLA system. These include multiple sclerosis, coeliac disease, and various skin complaints.

Two disorders associated with HLA are interesting because they are fundamentally unlike the others: hemachromatosis, a metabolic defect that affects the liver (and other organs) and is not an inflammatory condition, and narcolepsy, a strange condition of unknown cause in which, from time to time, people have a pathological tendency to fall asleep.

We find a curious discrepancy in the relations among arthritis, HLA molecules, and different types of infection. All of the theory and experimental work on animals suggests that there is a possible link between HLA and viruses, and that this connection might apply especially to class I HLA molecules. Surprisingly, so far we have found no evidence of such an association in humans. People with particular HLA molecules have not been shown to be more susceptible to any type of viral arthritis, except the reactive arthritis associated with AIDS.

B27 itself is associated with reactive arthritis following bacterial infection with several different organisms, and with the reactive arthritis seen in people with AIDS. Furthermore, B27 seems to be associated with the reactive arthritis seen with parasite infections. But rheumatic fever does not have a simple association with B27 or any other HLA molecule. (Although one report suggests a more complicated link with HLA, this association has not been confirmed.) We now know that erythema nodosum and its arthritis are associated with both a class I and a class II molecule in sarcoidosis, but it has not yet been established whether similar associations occur with other causes of erythema nodosum. Finally, in the spirochete infection in Lyme disease, the HLA association is not with the frequency of disease but with its severity. In summary, the strongest human association so far is between HLA and the remnants of dead organisms, especially certain strains of several varieties of bacteria.

From the early days of HLA and disease, those of us who were conducting research on this relationship have constituted an informal club. Whatever our individual interests, we follow carefully the advances in all of the other diseases associated with the genetics of HLA, T-cell receptor, or antibody molecules. Because the arthritic diseases provide the best models to date, what we learn about arthritis may well help us to discover and understand crucial, unknown aspects of common diseases as diverse as multiple sclerosis, psoriasis, narcolepsy, thyroiditis, and juvenile diabetes.

19

DNA, RNA, and Proteins

Medical science has been transformed in recent years by knowledge based on the fundamental process by which DNA (deoxyribonucleic acid) makes RNA (ribonucleic acid), and RNA makes protein (see Figure 19). The consequent changes in research are so marked and so far-reaching that it would be impossible to appreciate the latest advances in the study of arthritis without first returning to genetics. Later, we will consider the fascinating methods for investigating DNA, RNA, and protein molecules, the supreme importance of which will be apparent in the chapters that follow. This book would be incomplete without a bit of the flavor of the sophisticated techniques now available.

When people think of genes, many of them imagine that their function is confined to the specialized reproductive cells, the sperm and the ovum, which pass on the instructions for the creation of a new individual. Therefore, it is essential to emphasize that the function of genes continues in almost all cells throughout life, quite apart from the need to provide more reproductive cells for the next generation.

The nucleus of every cell in our body contains DNA, but the incredible library of information in the DNA is useless unless the messages are passed on to make proteins. Consider a hypothetical situation in which the DNA for a new cell has been provided but the exquisite detail of the cell's structure has not yet developed. How does the DNA perform the seemingly impossible task of equipping this miniature factory? The answer is that the DNA constructs a team of messengers called RNA that is dispatched to the part of the cytoplasm (outside the nucleus) where proteins form.

Proteins are of fundamental importance because they control the chemical processes of life. Among their many functions they provide structural support, enzymes, transport, messengers, and receptors. HLA molecules, T-cell receptor molecules, and antibody molecules, essential elements in our story, are all proteins.

The function of these complicated molecules depends primarily on the arrangement of their three-dimensional structures. Each protein molecule is made up of numerous building blocks, called *amino acids*, that are connected in line. In turn, each amino acid comprises ten to twenty-seven atoms. A typical protein is the hemoglobin molecule, made up of ten thousand atoms.

Genes (the functional units of heredity and protein synthesis) are arranged along microscopic thread-like structures called *chromosomes*. Every nucleus in each of our cells contains at least fifty thousand genes in a set of twenty-three pairs of chromosomes. The word "genome" means a complete set of chromosomes (and, therefore, of genes). As all biology students learn in school, a chromosome is composed of a long thread of DNA in the form of a double helix, with two intertwined strands of phosphate and sugar connected at regular intervals by cross-struts made of bases. The basic building block of DNA, containing a phosphate, a sugar, and a base, is called a *nucleotide*.

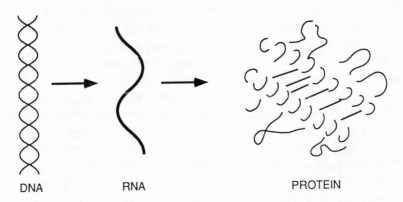

DNA   RNA   PROTEIN

Figure 19 • The process of DNA making RNA, and RNA making protein.

Approximately 3 trillion nucleotides reside in each cell (providing a set of 1 trillion instructions). Despite this huge number, there are only four types of nucleotides—usually referred to by the abbreviations of their chemical names as A (adenine), C (cytosine), G (guanine), and T (thymine). The genetic code is the sequence in which these letters are written—in groups of three.

The nucleotides in one molecule, if placed in their double helix form, would constitute an extremely thin structure more than a meter long. So the packing of this molecule inside the tiny nucleus is an incredible feat. To achieve sufficient miniaturization, each double helix is neatly folded in elaborate coiled structures called *nucleosomes*, which in turn are formed into *loops*. Because a human being is made up of many cells, his or her DNA molecules, laid end to end, would encircle the world several times.

One of the marvels of cell division is that this lengthy DNA uncoils within a particular nucleus, duplicates, separates, and is repackaged in two new nuclei without getting entangled. The two complementary strands of the double helix act as templates to direct the synthesis of the identical new pair of strands; the whole process is controlled by many enzymes and other proteins.

When a strand of DNA passes its message to a parallel strand of RNA, the sequence of nucleotides is transcribed from the DNA to the RNA, using a code in which the bases have the same number but a slightly different identity. The messenger RNA carrying the code migrates to the cytoplasm to initiate the production of a protein. There the sequence of bases on the RNA is translated into twenty types of amino acids, with three bases providing the instructions for making one amino acid. Then, in an elaborate process not yet fully understood, the amino acids (still in a straight line) are folded into the three-dimensional shape that is so important to a protein's function.

Since fifty thousand genes reside in a cell, all expressing their identity by the formation of proteins, it is inevitable that many of their messages are integrated within the cytoplasm. As a simple example, often one gene creates a structure and another gene regulates its function. Furthermore, cooperating genes need not be from the same chromosome. Genes from two chromosomes are required to create a molecule of hemoglobin, and genes from three chromosomes are needed to form antibodies or T-cell receptors.

If a protein molecule is broken down (degraded)—either in life within the body or in laboratory studies outside the body—it loses its intricate three-dimensional structure, as a knitted woolen garment does when unraveled. The molecule may also be broken into fragments called *peptides,* comprising only short chains of amino acids. In this simpler form, the sequence of amino acids in a peptide can be worked out in the laboratory, like identifying a series of marks on strands of wool. The entire sequence of amino acids in a protein can also be determined.

As a consequence of advances in laboratory techniques, tasks that previously seemed impossible or that took many years to perform can now be completed in hours.

- DNA can be extracted from the nuclei of cells, usually from polymorphs or lymphocytes in the blood. Specific enzymes (called *restriction nucleases*) are then used to divide the DNA at precise locations. This technique makes it easy to cut the DNA on either side of the part that one wants to study. The resulting segment can be separated and analyzed in detail.
- Because DNA comprises a chain of nucleotides, all in a line, the sequence of the bases in that chain can be identified. The process has been automated to such an extent that the sequence of nucleotides can be recorded at the rate of twenty-four thousand pairs of bases a day. Because that is still not fast enough, new apparatus is being designed to speed the process.
- Using a technique called the *polymerase chain reaction* (commonly known as PCR), selected segments of DNA can be multiplied several million times in a test tube within a few hours.
- In DNA cloning, a segment of DNA is spliced into the DNA of bacteria. The bacteria undergo rapid multiplication by their customary cell division and produce protein. This is the basis of genetic engineering, in which the DNA segment is altered before it is inserted into the bacteria. The result: new or especially desired proteins.
- When the sequence of the nucleotides in a segment of DNA has been worked out, the protein produced by that part of the DNA can be predicted with the aid of a computer.
- There are three ways of making gene probes: from a segment of DNA, from a segment of RNA, or from a segment of a solitary strand of DNA (made by persuading a segment of RNA to transcribe its sequence onto a complementary strand of DNA). Each of these probes can be made readily identifiable by attaching chemical markers at

specific locations on each segment. Armed with these probes, we can study cells or tissues. Each probe seeks out any identical small segment of DNA or RNA, and the markers reveal the presence of minute quantities of genetic material. Thus, we can establish which elements of DNA and RNA are active in producing which proteins at a given time.

- The sequence of the amino acids in part of a protein can be determined by commercially available automatic machines. This process has many uses in research.
- Once the sequence of a protein is known, we can deduce with a high degree of accuracy the sequence of nucleotides in the DNA from which it is derived.
- Proteins can be constructed in automatic apparatus. Even some of the sophisticated receptors and other features of the immune system have been manufactured.

Remarkable as these techniques may be, we must never forget the limitations of investigating proteins by unraveling them and then studying peptide chains in only two dimensions. An intact protein is approximately spherical in shape and does not function as a chain. Although it is helpful to know the sequence of amino acids in a protein chain, theoretically amino acids can be oriented in space and joined by cross-links in an infinite number of ways. When the detailed structure is known, amino acids that appear to be far apart in a linear chain may in three dimensions be joined to form a critical functioning unit.

To understand proteins more fully, it is often essential to determine their three-dimensional structure, as we saw in Rosalind Franklin's work on DNA using x-ray analysis. So it is enlightening to step back from the modern technology of proteins, DNA, and RNA to look at the emergence of x-ray analysis early in this century and then to consider the technology now used in resolving the structure of proteins.

Everyone is familiar with the ability of x-rays to pass through dense structures such as bone, but this property of x-rays is not what makes them invaluable in the investigation of proteins. The feature that determines their use in the study of atoms and molecules is the small size of the waves they form.

The investigation of minute objects requires minute waves. Light waves, at 20,000 waves to the centimeter, have far too large an amplitude to "see" an atom's structure: a light wave is in the same proportion to an atom as a camel to the eye of a needle. Because the waves are too big to oscillate within an atom, light waves pass through without being altered. No matter how much you magnify with a microscope the light waves emerging from an atom or molecule, you will still be unable to see their structures in detail. The solution is to resort to waves 1/10,000 the length of light waves—x-rays. X-rays enable us to see things thousands of times smaller than we can see with the best light microscope.

There are problems, however. A single atom cannot be studied, because the x-rays would destroy it before anything could be recorded. We need to examine large numbers of identical atoms or molecules, all oriented in the same direction. This requires a crystal—in which, by definition, there is a systematic lattice arrangement of atoms and molecules, with plane faces intersecting at definite angles to give the crystal its characteristic symmetry.

It was Max von Laue, working at the University of Munich in the department of the famous Wilhelm Conrad Röntgen, who posed the question that initiated this type of investigation. He knew that atoms in crystals have a regular arrangement, and that the distance between those atoms in a crystal is about ten-millionths of a millimeter. He also knew that this was approximately the wavelength of an x-ray. So he asked whether, when x-rays are passed through a crystal, they might give rise to interference phenomena.

Röntgen was skeptical and disinterested, but two assistants in the laboratory agreed to gamble on a long shot. They put a copper sulfate crystal in the beam of an x-ray and attempted to record the reflection by placing a photographic plate in front of the crystal. Nothing happened, and they almost abandoned the project. Then one of them had the idea that he should put the plate on the crystal's far side. To their delight, not only did the main beam register, but spots were seen that had been scattered in an orderly fashion due to deflection by the crystal. Interference in the crystal had evidently split the x-ray beam into several small beams. Also, as the crystal was rotated, the beam would flash at a certain angle. Because a crystal is not flat like a mirror but is a series of planes, each plane caused a separate flash. For his research, in 1914 von Laue won the Nobel Prize.

X-ray analysis was taken up by many people, but especially by two Englishmen, William Henry Bragg (1862–1942) and his son, William Lawrence Bragg (1890–1971), then a student at Cambridge. The Braggs' first contribution was the x-ray spectrometer. A crystal could be placed in this instrument in such a way that it reflected an x-ray beam in any direction, and the strength of the beam could be measured in an ionization chamber. Using this technique, the elder Bragg soon found that each metal used as a source of radiation gave a characteristic x-ray spectrum of a definite wavelength. The various faces of crystals could be examined, and it was possible to deduce the way atoms were arranged in sheets. After a year of concentrated work, the Braggs had established the structures of fluorspar, cuprite, zinc blende, iron pyrites, sodium nitrate, the calcite group of minerals, potassium chloride, sodium chloride, and diamonds.

It was an exciting time. Years later the son, Lawrence, wrote: "It was like discovering an alluvial gold field with nuggets lying around waiting to be picked up . . . It was a glorious time, when we worked far into every night with new worlds unfolding before us in the silent laboratory." Then came 1914, and for Lawrence the end of research until after World War I. In 1915 his father made the important proposal that x-ray measurements should be interpreted as part of a Fourier series (the harmonic components of a complex periodic wave); this proposal was later improved and adopted as a standard method of presenting x-ray results. In the same year, both Braggs won the Nobel Prize. Subsequently they became Sir William and Sir Lawrence.

Years later, Sir Lawrence compared crystal analysis to solving a very difficult crossword puzzle:

Each structure that has been analysed has told us something about the way atoms are arranged, such as the amount of space each kind of atom takes up in the structure, what neighbouring atoms it is likely to be associated with, how they are likely to be grouped around it, and so forth. Knowing this one can make intelligent guesses when tackling a new structure, trying out various likely arrangements till the glorious moment arrives when everything fits in. Any symmetry the crystal possesses is of considerable assistance. Still, with all these aids, structure analysis is an arduous task. Those of us who began in the early days and grew up with it acquired our skill and patience by stages. We would live with a single structure ever in our minds for perhaps a year, with tentative pictures of it before us when we were shaving in the morning and at our meals, and dreaming of it at night, till finally something clicked and the answer came.

Following the impetus provided by the Braggs, the determination of structure by the use of x-ray crystallography flourished in England, especially in London and in Manchester. For a while, with no equals elsewhere in the world, a band of outstanding scientists carried out a series of intricate investigations, gradually tackling substances of greater and greater complexity.

We now meet two institutions that challenged this temporary British supremacy: Caltech and Linus Pauling. The California Institute of Technology began in 1891 as a school of arts in Pasadena called the Throop Polytechnic Institute. By 1910 it had become a College of Technology, and plans were made to move to a green field site southeast of town. The name California Institute of Technology was introduced in 1920 and immediately shortened to Caltech. From the beginning, the new institute had two special advantages: it was richly endowed by wealthy local people, and it succeeded in attracting many eminent scientists.

Linus Pauling was born in Portland, Oregon, in 1901 and grew up in cowboy country, where his father ran a drugstore. Pauling obtained a degree as a chemical engineer from Oregon Agricultural College and in 1922 went to Caltech. There he began a thirty-year program of building a strong school of structural crystallography. For many years there was friendly competition between Caltech and Britain, particularly Cambridge.

The younger institution soon showed that it had the advantages of a fresh approach and a willingness to adopt new techniques. Bolstered by recent concepts of quantum mechanics and realizing the importance of distances between atoms, Pauling was well aware of the limitations and problems of x-ray techniques. During a visit to Ludwigshaven, Germany, he saw electron diffraction apparatus in use for the first time. He was so impressed that when he returned to Caltech, he arranged for a similar apparatus to be built there. Soon afterward he began to investigate amino acids and peptides, with the apparent long-term goal of working out the structure of proteins. In 1950 he shook the world of crystallography when he was the first to report the helical structure of certain proteins. It was Pauling who laid the foundations of understanding alpha helices, gamma helices, beta sheets, and other structures within protein molecules.

One of Pauling's greatest feats was his work on chemical bonds, atomic distances, and bond directions in complicated structures. Indeed, it was for this research that he won the 1954 Nobel Prize in chemistry. Six years later he won the Nobel Peace Prize for his campaign against nuclear weapons. Without doubt, he is one of the most distinguished chemists of all time.

As an aside, for those who take an interest in the workings of the mind, Pauling's personal experience with problem solving is intriguing. Many people wonder why ideas come to them when they are relaxed or asleep, and why rough plans become altered and refined after sleeping on them. Somehow, original thoughts flourish on the subconscious level, presumably because they are less inhibited. Pauling deliberately took advantage of this useful process by reviewing in his mind, just before going to sleep, the problems he had not settled during an active day. Often he found that the solutions would be apparent when he awoke.

Another person to undertake the seemingly impossible task of determining the structure of proteins was John Desmond Bernal, working in the Cavendish Laboratory at Cambridge. The son of an Irish Catholic farmer, he became an ardent communist in his undergraduate years at Cambridge. With long, untidy hair and a striking appearance, he embodied the image of genius and was nicknamed "Sage" because of the remarkable breadth of his knowledge.

At first, all attempts to obtain x-rays of protein crystals were unsuccessful. Bernal's observation that the crystals must be kept wet was crucial. This finding led him to mount the crystals in small silicon tubes, sealed at each end. The first x-ray of a protein crystal was published in 1934 by Bernal and Dorothy Hodgkin (who in 1968 won the Nobel Prize for her elucidation of the structure of penicillin and vitamin B_{12}).

Bernal was joined by Max Perutz, who, as a graduate student, decided to tackle the incredibly intricate structure of hemoglobin—at a time when the most complicated structure that investigators had resolved had only fifty-eight atoms. Perutz's project took twenty-three years! Ten years after he started, Perutz was joined by John (later Sir John) Kendrew, who took on the structure of myoglobin (a key protein in muscles that is about one-quarter the size of hemoglobin). For their contributions Perutz and Kendrew won the Nobel Prize in 1962.

One of the most difficult problems the two men encountered was the determination of phases. The spots on the x-ray films indicated the wavelength and amplitude of the waves they were studying, but not their phases. Perutz adopted a technique that had been used for investigating simpler crystals, whereby heavy metals such as mercury and gold were affixed to the crystals as markers. The addition of a metal altered the x-ray pattern without materially changing the protein's shape. Although one metal compound alone did not resolve the riddle of the phases, the use of several metals was invaluable. Perutz and Kendrew determined the phase by comparing x-ray plates of the protein molecule with other x-ray plates taken after a number of metals had been added to the protein molecule.

At the beginning of their research activities, they lacked suitable computers to analyze their data. They were fortunate, though, that computers became available at exactly the right time. Kendrew pioneered their use in analyzing protein structure, but even then the process was re markably complicated. It seems unbelievable now that, when analyzing a three-dimensional shape, they had to erect a host of steel rods in a model six feet in diameter and use colored clips to represent points of high electron density. As a result, the helices showed up as spirals of colored clips. Since that time x-ray analysis has become far more automated. Recording can be done by electronic detectors, and the computers that analyze the results are vastly more powerful and versatile.

20

The Beauty of Crystals

Every few years, when the results of a research study are announced, people say, "So that's the answer, at last." Or, "Surely that team will get a Nobel Prize." Such was the response in 1987 when Jack Strominger, Don Wiley, Pamela Bjorkman, and their colleagues reported that they had used x-ray crystallography to determine the structure of an HLA molecule. This work ranks as one of the outstanding advances in the history of medicine, and in due course it will come to be seen as the double helix of arthritis—and one of the keys to future knowledge.

Jack Strominger is a biochemist working in the Department of Biochemistry and Molecular Biology at Harvard University. In the course of his distinguished career, Strominger has made many discoveries related to subjects in biochemistry, immunology, and genetics, including the mechanism of the action of penicillin and the detailed structures of bacteria, viruses, and T-cell receptors. Like others in our story, he has a genius for taking leaps of faith and seeing what others cannot see.

Don Wiley works independently in the same department and has similar broad interests. His best-known previous research was on the structure of a molecule related to the influenza virus. He has also investigated the structure and function of parasites and is an authority on crystallography.

The initial step in studying a molecule of HLA is to isolate it in pure form. This procedure was attempted first by Arnold Sanderson at the Queen Victoria Hospital in East Grinstead, England—famous for its surgical treatment of RAF airmen during World War II. As Sanderson reported in *Nature* in 1964 and 1968, he succeeded in separating HLA substances from human spleens. In retrospect, it is clear that his methods would have resulted in a satisfactory degree of purification, but at the time he had neither the techniques to prove it nor the facilities to attain adequate levels of purification. Instead, he generously passed on all he knew about HLA to his friend Jack Strominger. As Sanderson told me, he knew that Harvard would gallop away from East Grinstead, but he was only too happy to applaud.

The subsequent investigations of the molecular structure of HLA led to spectacular results that have established Strominger as one of the undisputed world leaders in the field. He had what Sanderson lacked: a large department filled with brilliant scientists, financial resources, and a plentiful supply of cells in culture (obviously a better source of HLA molecules than a crude extract of tissue from spleens). Strominger's work also coincided with the revolution in gene technology.

A group of British scientists, including some excellent people from East Grinstead, went to work in Strominger's laboratory, and by 1973 they had purified HLA molecules from a culture of special cells donated by a person living in an Indiana Amish community. These cells contained twenty times as many HLA molecules as do the cells in human spleens. Using their technique, published in 1975 with Sanderson as co-author, Strominger's team managed to harvest 3 to 4 milligrams of molecules from every 100 grams of cells. Although this does not sound like much, according to Strominger it was the beginning of their success. Everything flowed from that point, including even more elegant methods of purification.

Members of Strominger's department then worked out the amino acid sequence in a typical HLA molecule, and they learned two valuable facts. First, the structure of an HLA molecule is similar to that of an antibody molecule, including amino acid sequences that are common to both. Second, the HLA molecule has two main components: a large one derived from the sixth chromosome and a small one derived from the fifteenth chromosome. From this, the team gradually added pieces of the HLA molecular structure. DNA cloning (by using antibodies to screen libraries of genes in human lymphocytes and then growing clones in *E. coli*, a common type of bacteria) enabled the researchers to alter the molecule, one amino acid at a time, and determine how this affected the molecule's function.

From these painstaking techniques, a picture of the HLA molecule emerged. But everyone, especially Wiley and Strominger, had known from the beginning that the ultimate objective was to determine the structure of the molecule by using x-ray diffraction techniques. The essence of crystallography is that the three-dimensional structure of a molecule is often the principal clue to understanding how it works.

Readers unfamiliar with the way research operates today may not appreciate the extent to which success depends on collaboration between young graduate students and the heads of departments or other senior staff who supervise the investigation. The graduates do the hands-on work in the laboratory, read the literature, and make many of the critical decisions because of their day-to-day involvement. The seniors know the field, have extensive experience, and are available for advice. As you can imagine, the way this works in practice varies, often making it impossible for outsiders to apportion credit for what is done. In this instance, though, the teamwork was perfectly balanced.

In what follows, I have elected to tell the story of the determination of the crystal structure of the HLA molecule from Pamela Bjorkman's point of view. I particularly wish to illustrate the essential contribution of young scientists. After all, the future of research belongs to the young. Bjorkman now heads her own laboratory at Caltech, where she hopes to offer her graduate students projects as interesting and important as the HLA molecule—although she admits that her own opportunity will be hard to beat.

Looking back at the eight years she spent determining the crystal structure of the HLA molecule, Bjorkman responded to my many questions in a long letter explaining what had happened and how she felt about the events at the time. Her account, which I have shortened slightly, provides insight into the courage, persistence, and dedication of young scientists.

> I'll preface this letter by saying that it is, of course, my version of things, and that is necessarily the viewpoint of a graduate student, since that is what I was during most of this work.
>
> I was fortunate to be in the right place at the right time. The Strominger lab had been characterizing HLA for ten years before I tried to crystallize it; if they hadn't worked out a purification procedure, we would never have a structure today. Jack and his lab laid the groundwork for a crystallographer to step in and solve the structure. When I first started, I was a student learning crystallography, so I was lucky to

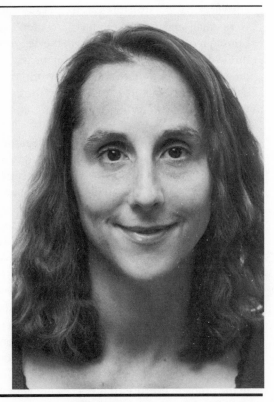

Pamela Bjorkman. As a graduate student working with professors Don Wiley and Jack Strominger at Harvard University, Bjorkman was the first to work out the three-dimensional structure of an HLA molecule.

have the chance to learn it from Don and the people in his lab while working on such an interesting structure. Being in his lab instilled in me the idea that it wasn't enough to solve a crystal structure, one had to go on to use the structural information to understand how it worked.

One person who had a huge impact on the completion of the structure was Anastasia Haykov ("Nastia"), who did hundreds of protein purifications over many years. Since the yield of protein was so low, she prepared material every time we had enough cells. On average this worked out to be about every two weeks. I was also privileged to work with Bill Bennett, Boudjema Samraoui, and Mark Saper, all postdoctoral fellows who contributed in many ways to the final structure determination.

The structure took a long time to finish—eight years, actually. People often ask me why it took so long and what I did all that time. The short answer is that the structure was technically difficult because the crystals were small and few in number; I couldn't grow them reproducibly. Consequently, all the usual steps in the determination of a crystal structure—data collection, searching for heavy atom derivatives, and so on—simply took longer and didn't work as well as they would have done if the crystals had been larger. During those eight years, there were numerous times when I thought that the structure would never be solved.

After hearing Don Wiley talk at a departmental retreat, I got very excited about crystallography and decided to rotate in his laboratory in hopes that I could work on the crystal structure of a membrane protein. Don was working on the influenza virus hemagglutinin structure at the time, but was very interested in the image reconstruction techniques recently used by Richard Henderson and Nigel Unwin. So Don taught me about image reconstruction and electron microscopy; and I tried to make two-dimensional ordered arrays of hemagglutinin and virus proteins for low-angle x-ray scattering work.

At about that time Jim Kaufman, a senior graduate student in the Strominger lab, suggested that I try to crystallize HLA. They had milligram amounts of pure protein which had been solubilized by papain cleavage from cell membranes. I then found out how much protein the Strominger lab had and how pure it was before I asked Don if I could work in his lab on HLA as a thesis project. Originally, I was interested in the problem because HLA is a cell membrane protein. Now, like others, I think that that aspect of HLA is probably its least interesting feature.

Naturally, it had already occurred to Jack Strominger and to Don that someone should try to crystallize HLA, but the project had never gotten off the ground. A few years previously, Peter Parham (at that time a post-doc in Jack's lab) had purified some HLA and given it to Don, but the sample was lost during a concentration step and no one ever actually tried to crystallize it.

When I told Don that I wanted to work on HLA, he agreed that it would be an interesting crystal structure to study but didn't think it was an appropriate project for a graduate student, because if it didn't work, I wouldn't have anything to write a thesis about. Eventually, after a bit of persuasion on my part, he said that I could work on HLA for the summer but we wouldn't call it a thesis project until it was clear it would work. He also advised me to pick another subject as a back-up in case the HLA never crystallized.

I then made a formal arrangement to be a joint graduate student in the Wiley and Strominger labs. As a back-up project, I decided I would work on monitoring transmembrane signaling by HLA, using a cytoplasmic fluorescent probe, but I ended up doing very little work on that project because the HLA protein crystallized under the first conditions that I tried.

Don showed me how to set up precipitation trials to see where the protein precipitated with various salts. He also showed me how to set up crystallization trays. Because we didn't have much protein, I tried to dissolve the precipitated protein by resuspending it on a coverslip over a reservoir with a low concentration of PEG [polyethylene glycol]. After a week had gone by, I looked at the crystallization trays, but there were no crystals. By chance I happened to look at the drop precipitated with PEG in which I was trying to recover protein for crystallization trials; and there were some crystals. Apparently they had formed while the protein was going back into solution. They were not single crystals and were small and thin, but they did diffract x-rays.

We never had much HLA protein to work with. Each preparation took two weeks and yielded only 2 to 4 milligrams from 200 liters of cells. Then, disappointingly, the source of cells was cut off for over a year. I spent that year trying various ways to improve the crystals. Eventually, I could grow single crystals of HLA-A2 and HLA-Aw68 sometimes, but not reproducibly. These crystals were very small and only grew if they were seeded with crystalline nuclei.

I spent quite a while trying to collect diffraction data using our laboratory x-ray sets, but the crystals were so small and thin that the diffraction patterns took too long to record. Protein crystals have only a finite life in the x-ray beam, so that I could get only a few usable diffraction patterns from each crystal. Also, the crystals were so thin and difficult to handle that I broke many of them while they were being mounted.

After much disappointment, we decided to use synchrotron radiation as our x-ray source because it is more intense and more suitable in the study of small crystals. Protein crystals die due to radiation decay, which is believed to be time dependent, so that a high-intensity beam used for a short time produces more data than a weaker beam used for a long time. When investigating HLA crystals, we could obtain ten times as much information using synchrotron radiation than using x-rays from a rotating anode in our lab. As we had only a very small number of single crystals, synchrotron x-rays meant the difference between being able to collect data from HLA crystals or not collecting data.

The problem was that the nearest available source of synchrotron radiation was at Hamburg in Germany. On our first trip there, we collected a complete set of data from only two crystals! Over a period of years I traveled to Hamburg seven times, trips which I found very exciting because I had never been to Europe before. It was always amazing to see beautiful diffraction patterns resulting from these tiny crystals after having spent two years trying to collect data using the x-ray sources in the lab.

On most of the trips to Germany, I was helped by Bill Bennett, a postdoc fellow in Don's lab. He is an excellent crystallographer and taught me a lot about data collection and processing of films. To analyze the x-ray films, it is necessary to measure the intensity of each reflection and assign it an index. This is done by computer programs which take into account the space group of the crystal and its orientation in the beam. I often came home from a synchrotron trip with a thousand films to analyze, so I spent a lot of time doing what crystallographers call "film scanning" and "data reduction."

This period of the work took a long time because I couldn't find any useful "heavy-atom derivatives." As you know, derived crystals are used to provide information about the phases of the diffracted x-ray waves, which, with the intensity of the waves, are used to calculate electron density maps. The intensities are easily measured on the films, but all information about the phases of each reflection is lost. In order to approximate phases, one adds a heavy metal to the protein, preferably in one or two defined places, and then collects the diffraction data again. Intensity differences between the new data and the old data can then be used to approximate the phases.

In theory one needs at least two unique derivatives to determine the phases unambiguously, but in practice more are often necessary. After checking over a hundred compounds, I ended up with fourteen from which I collected some data but only one that produced useful phases. The screening for derivatives and the data collection from derivatives went on for many years. This sort of story is typical in protein crystallography. Whenever there's a problem, it's almost always due to poor derivatives.

After my going to Germany for a year or so, the synchrotrons at Cornell in New York and Stanford near San Francisco became available for use by protein crystallographers. Since Cornell was closer, I started going there; in all, I went there more times than I can remember. The low point of the entire HLA project was during a trip to the Cornell synchrotron. I took a year's worth of crystals to screen for derivatives.

Unfortunately, there was something wrong with the x-ray camera; by the time I figured that out, the crystals were already mounted and had been exposed to the beam, making them unsuitable for further use. I didn't get a single diffraction pattern and the production of crystals for an entire year was wasted.

Trips to synchrotrons were never much fun. The synchrotrons are usually run by high-energy physicists doing collision experiments; they often turn off the synchrotron x-ray beam without warning to alter parameters in their own experiments. Thus, one never knew when the beam would be on. So when there was a beam, I had to work continuously until it went down again, resulting in many nights without sleep. Worse than that was when the beam went down unexpectedly, usually announced as a small problem that would be remedied immediately. I once spent five days at Cornell waiting for a beam that was always due to come on in one hour.

At some point it seemed as though I would never get a second useful derivative, so I decided to try to do what I could with the single one I had, using many techniques familiar to crystallographers. After many attempts I saw something that was the size and shape of part of an immunoglobulin. It is hard to describe what seeing this in the map was like. It doesn't sound much, but it was the first indication that I was on the right track. Then I found some more features that looked like protein. They were definitely there, although the map was very noisy. I remember being far too nervous to look through the rest of the map, so I went home for a few hours before I had the courage to look at the map some more. Then, when I came back, I couldn't make any sense out of the rest of the map.

The HLA map was never of high quality because it was calculated with a single derivative and because the data that went into it weren't great as a result of the small size of the crystals. At that time, despite being a crystallographer for six years, I had no experience of tracing electron density maps of any quality because I hadn't got the HLA crystals to that stage yet. I tried tracing "good" maps calculated from other proteins, such as antibodies, and that too was extremely difficult. Then Boudjema Samraoui joined Don's lab as a post-doc fellow. He had been at Oxford and had a lot of experience tracing electron density maps. Somehow, he found another immunoglobulin-like structure and some helical regions. So we decided to try a different procedure in which you build as much structure into the map as you can, then use the partial model to calculate phases which are combined with your observed phases. After that you should be able to build a little more, calculate more phases to make a new map, into which you build more of the structure. And so on. I tried many different schemes; we went through many cycles of model building followed by map calculation. The whole procedure always worried me because it is subject to a lot of bias, so I tried various ways to reduce the bias inherent in the procedure.

After a year of these calculations, what resulted was a partial model, complete in some respects and incomplete in others. We could see two long helices and the eight-stranded pleated sheet, but I couldn't see how the individual strands and helices were connected to one another. Most puzzling was a long piece of electron density that didn't seem connected to anything and ran down the middle of the site.

During this time, I'd gotten my Ph.D. with a very technical thesis that didn't show much of biological interest. By then I'd been working on HLA for seven years, and it was time to move on to another lab. I decided to move to Stanford because the person who later became my husband had already moved to Stanford the year before and we didn't want to live on opposite sides of the country for very long. Also, my father (who lived in Oregon) was ill, and it would be easier to visit him from California.

For all these reasons, I made arrangements to go to Mark Davis' lab at Stanford to try to make soluble T-cell receptors suitable for crystallization. But I didn't want to stop working on HLA before I saw what it looked like, so I stayed in Don's lab as a post-doc. As you can imagine, the structure had become somewhat of an obsession with me, and I didn't want to stop working on it when it was so close to being finished. I had spent most of my adult life working on that crystal structure, and I felt I would never be satisfied, scientifically or otherwise, if I didn't finish it.

By the summer of 1986, I had the problem that everything except HLA was pulling me away from Harvard and toward Stanford. Don realized this and he also knew about my obsession with the structure, although not entirely approving. Finally, he said that I could go to Stanford and finish the HLA structure there, since from then on it was all computer work that could be done anywhere. This was a very generous thing for him to do, and I have always appreciated it. Mark Davis kindly agreed that I could do the computer work on HLA at Stanford, while trying to learn molecular biology and make soluble T-cell receptor.

I then tried another approach to finish the structure. Seven years before, I had grown a second crystal form of HLA in which the molecules were packed differently, but I could never get enough of them to use for data collection. These crystals were all grown by the laborious technique of washing a single crystal and then using it as a seed in a fresh solution of protein. I had taught this technique to Nastia, and she had spent a lot of time making crystals of the second type. Fortunately, the crystals in the second form were a bit larger, and eventually I had enough to collect data.

Having the data from the second crystals meant that I could calculate a new electron density map that was entirely independent of the first one and if I could determine the position of the HLA molecule in the new map, I could average the electron densities in the two maps. The technique of averaging is a very powerful method of phase improvement used by protein crystallographers. The problem was finding the orientation that related the molecules in the two maps. I used a six-dimensional searching algorithm on the computer. The program took the partial model from the first map and placed it on a grid point in the second map. It rotated and translated the model (through three rotation angles and three translation directions) until it found the best fit. The program took a whole week of computer time.

I ran the program several times without success, so I made a trivial adjustment to the new map and ran the program again—without expecting any good results. A week later, I couldn't believe it when I saw there was a huge peak at one place in the map. By visual inspection I could see it was right. To me this was the happiest time of the whole structure determination. I knew then that we could average the two maps and finish the structure. I kept wanting to tell people about the results and show them the map, but nobody at Stanford was a crystallographer, so they didn't understand what I was so excited about.

After getting a lot of advice from Don, I set up the procedure to do the averaging of the two maps. This is a cyclical procedure and very labor intensive. Mark Saper had just gone to Don's lab to work on HLA, so I went back to Harvard to show him the first averaged map and to talk about how to do the rest of the averaging. Mark did the remainder of the averaging cycles, working out methods on the way to optimize the procedure to make the best final electron density map. A few months later (May 1987), when Mark had a map that we thought was promising, I flew back to Harvard so we could try to trace the remainder. In five days we finished the rest of the structure that had been unconnected for over a year. Then what we had suspected for a few months was confirmed: the piece of electron density that ran through the middle was not part of the HLA molecule. It represented something else—probably a peptide.

Once the chain was traced, I went back to Stanford and we wrote the two *Nature* papers in two months. Those two months were the highlight of my scientific career and probably always will be because it was so much fun locating all the interesting sites on the molecule since they were all in such obvious places. Those that were polymorphic all pointed in toward the peptide-binding site, and so did those that affected T-cell recognition. I gathered up as many papers as I could about HLA molecules and we could almost always interpret the data using the HLA structure. It was fun to think about these things because at that time we had the HLA structure to ourselves, as no one else had seen it yet.

It was hard to squeeze everything we wanted to say into the two *Nature* papers. The strange thing about those papers for me is that they represented only two months of work from the past eight years of my life. I had spent almost all of those years worrying about crystals, or technical details about data, phases, or electron density maps. None of that went into those papers—except a brief description of methods that I am sure nobody read.

When it was all finished, and at last I had the luxury of looking at the molecule, it all seemed so obvious that I didn't understand why someone hadn't figured it out before. I also felt a great relief that it was finally over. During those eight years, I had often wondered if I had been doing something fundamentally wrong so that the structure couldn't be solved. Now I could call myself a crystallographer because I had solved a structure.

You see, crystallography is a very different sort of science from most others. You really have done nothing until you are completely finished with a structure. I'd been without much to say to any biologist for eight years, and it wasn't easy to begin one's scientific career that way. But finishing the HLA structure was such an incredible reward that I felt privileged to have worked on it. The structure is truly an example to biologists of how three-dimensional structures aid in determining biological function. Suddenly there was a rational basis for so many things. I felt almost guilty because our structure was only interesting in light of the work of so many other laboratories.

Fortuitously, the HLA structure was finished at exactly the right time for it to be appreciated maximally. And the credit for its impact should go to the molecule itself, because its structure is so beautifully simplistic and easy to understand. I was incredibly lucky that I did the crystallography on a molecule whose structure ended up answering a lot of biological questions. I had sometimes feared that the structure would end up being boring, or somehow not revealing anything about how it works. But it is, I think, a very nice-looking molecule. I could have done the same work on a different molecule without such a revealing structure, and not be writing this letter to you today.

I probably think about the HLA structure differently from other people. I have certain favorite parts of the molecule because I remember what the electron density map looked like in that region. This is common among crystallographers who have worked on a structure for a long time. One thing that pleased me about the structure was that the way the molecules are packed in a crystal probably explains why I had so much trouble with thin crystals—due to a packing fault in the third dimension. I suppose no one else would find this interesting.

What Bjorkman, Wiley, Strominger, and their colleagues had demonstrated was a simple but sophisticated structure (Figure 20). The molecule they investigated is believed to be representative of all HLA molecules. The segments closest to the cell membrane are similar to segments of antibodies. On top of these is an eight-stranded sheet, upon which rest two long, helical regions. Between these helices lies the site where peptides bind. The two helical regions resemble complicated lips, while the eight-stranded sheet is like the back and sides of the mouth. Although Bjorkman is reluctant to be dogmatic, the mysterious, apparently unconnected fragment she mentions in her letter is believed to be an extraneous substance, presumably a peptide. It is this peptide within the groove that is presented to the equally sophisticated receptor of the T-cell.

Four years after the initial articles, in 1991 a further forward leap was signaled by a new report in *Nature:* Don Wiley and his colleagues at Harvard had determined the three-dimensional structure of HLA-B27. They had also studied a number of relevant peptides in the grooves of B27 molecules. Pockets were identified in the bottom and sides of the groove, capable of accommodating and binding peptides of several shapes. The way is now open for rapid progress in establishing the range of peptides that can bind to B27, with further details of how they are bound.

I can think of nothing more encouraging than the ability of Don

Wiley, Pamela Bjorkman, and others like them, to step inside the HLA molecule, to have a good look at its complicated structure, and to consider how peptides are handled there. Before long the detailed structure of T-cell receptor molecules will be known; presumably it will then be possible to study in three dimensions the interaction of HLA molecules, peptides, and T-cell receptors.

While these remarkable technical achievements continue, the contributions of clinicians must not be forgotten. We have known for several years that the HLA-B27 molecule is an integral part of the disease process of a number of disorders, and that when people who possess this

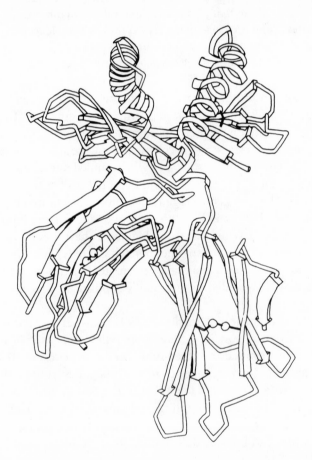

Figure 20 · The structure of an HLA molecule, as determined by Pamela Bjorkman and her colleagues.

molecule have certain bacterial infections, they are one hundred times more likely than others to develop arthritis three weeks later. All rheumatologists look forward to learning in what subtle ways the B27 molecule, the DR4 molecule, and other HLA molecules confer susceptibility to arthritis. By two different research techniques we know already that, in both HLA-DR4 and B27, five identified amino acids in the HLA molecule are critical in binding peptides. I have little doubt that the processing of antigens and the interaction between peptide, HLA molecule, and T-cell receptor molecule are crucial in the causation of most types of arthritis—and of similar common diseases.

21

Cells in Action

In arthritis research, two vexing questions linger: How do cells respond to antigens? How do cells assist the antigens to escape detection by scientists using the latest techniques? As we have noted before, microbes are seldom found in joints even when strong circumstantial evidence indicates that they are causing arthritis. Somehow this riddle must be solved.

At last we can appreciate why it is so important that Cohnheim studied the function of endothelial cells during inflammation, that Metchnikoff watched macrophages attack foreign substances, that Murphy championed lymphocytes, and that Dausset found the HLA system. During the eight years when Bjorkman was determining the structure of HLA molecules, our understanding of cell function was transformed.

I stated at the beginning of the book that inflammation can be caused by bacteria, viruses, parasites, noninfectious material, physical injury, local disease, foreign tissue, a normal part of the body in the wrong place, or a part of the body that has become abnormal. Later, when reviewing different types of arthritis, I mentioned fragments of dead bacteria and dead parasites, silica, vinyl chloride, toxic oil, organic solvents, drugs, paraffin, silicone, tobacco, asbestos, air pollution, and dietary protein. There is no reason to exclude any of those possibilities from our list of potential trigger factors. But for convenience I confine myself almost exclusively to proteins and fragments of proteins—that is, peptides.

Antigens can be divided into two types: those approaching cells from outside, and those formed within cells. Examples of the first type are fragments of bacteria that have entered the body from the environment. Examples of the second type are viruses that reproduce within cells and proteins that are made within cells. These external and internal antigens are handled in different ways, as we shall see.

Five types of cells are involved in arthritis: endothelial cells of the small blood vessels in the synovium, polymorphs, lymphocytes, dendritic cells, and macrophages.

Let us start with *endothelial cells.* In reviewing the means of access to joints, we noted that we always have a small proportion of foreign substances in our bloodstreams, and that the endothelial cells which line small blood vessels are critical in determining whether these substances invade the joints, especially after the small blood vessels have been damaged by inflammation. For a long time the overwhelming interest in cells of the immune system distracted attention from the sophisticated contribution of endothelial cells in initiating and perpetuating inflammation in arthritis. Within the past few years, though, we have seen far more research on how endothelial cells assist the passage of other cells, chemicals, and fluids from the bloodstream into the synovial tissues. Endothelial cells also take up foreign antigens from the bloodstream and present them to cells in the synovium for appropriate action. Many research groups today are studying means of treating arthritis by modifying the ease of access of antigens to the tissues within the joints.

Polymorphs are small, mobile cells with nuclei that take many shapes. You will remember that Metchnikoff discovered that these cells are avid phagocytes. In acute inflammation they act as shock troops in devouring foreign substances. Polymorphs are not thought to be involved primarily in diseases such as ankylosing spondylitis, reactive arthritis, psoriatic arthritis, and rheumatoid arthritis—but they are the most important cells when live bacteria or crystals are in the joints. In gout, polymorphs may become so engorged with crystals that they die and burst, releasing into the joint tissues and joint fluid enzymes that provoke severe inflammation and pain.

With *lymphocytes,* key cells in the immune system, a major step in our understanding was taken by Philip Gell of Birmingham, England, and Baruj Benacerraf, then at New York University, who in 1959 stimulated lymphocytes with proteins that were intact and with proteins that had been degraded. What we now call B-cells (B-lymphocytes) became blind and unresponsive when the protein had been degraded; that is, their response depended on recognizing the intact protein molecule's three-dimensional structure. By contrast, T-cells (T-lymphocytes) responded even when the protein had been degraded. This meant that, in some remarkable way, T-cells could identify sequences of amino acids in unraveled chains derived from protein molecules. Apart from this contrast in the recognition of proteins, B-cells and T-cells respond in different ways. As predicted by Behring, Kitasato, and Ehrlich, B-cells respond by producing antibodies, whereas T-cells muster a complicated and widespread cellular response. We now know that the antibody response of B-cells is far less specific than that of T-cells, which have a pivotal role in all specific responses.

Dendritic cells, similar to macrophages, may prove to be even more important in arthritis. So far there is definite evidence that dendritic cells can be more powerful than macrophages in stimulating inflammation, and preliminary evidence that they may transport foreign antigens from the site where they enter the body to the joints. But their role in arthritis has not yet been the subject of research as extensive as that on macrophages.

How *macrophages* (and other cells) prepare antigens for presentation to T-cells is fundamental in understanding cellular immunology. It is an example of the scientific process that four pieces of information became available from independent teams during a few months in 1973 and 1974. First, the groups in Westminster and Los Angeles found that HLA molecules are strongly associated with arthritis. Second, it was demonstrated that macrophages are dominant cells in rheumatoid arthritis and in the inflammatory response to silica. Third, it was shown that HLA molecules participate in the function of macrophages. And fourth, it was proved that T-cells recognize HLA molecules and foreign substances at the same time. For years, though, we did not put these facts together— nor did we understand the underlying mechanism that united the four discoveries.

Although many researchers have studied antigen processing by macrophages, Emil Unanue was a pioneer when he was at Harvard two decades ago, and he remains a prominent leader in this field. Unanue's first contribution was to extend Metchnikoff's investigation of the digestion of foreign substances by macrophages. His approach was to poison the cells in culture at discrete stages; in effect, he collected a series of time snapshots of what happened. His first finding was that a delay occurs after a macrophage and a foreign substance make contact and be-

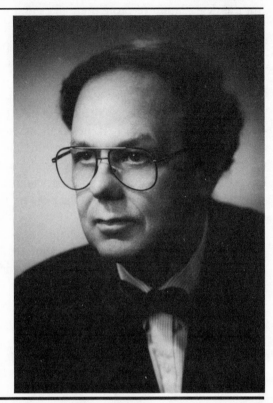

Emil Unanue. Working at Harvard University, Unanue pioneered the modern approach to the processing of foreign substances within cells. Now at Washington University in St. Louis, he continues to make important contributions in this rapidly advancing area.

fore presentation to a T-cell. The second finding was that energy is consumed during that delay. Both observations indicated an active process. It later transpired that T-cells cannot recognize most foreign substances unless they have first been processed by macrophages; the T-cells simply do not respond.

It was also learned that an object such as a bacterium or a protein is first bound to the surface of the macrophage, then internalized, then degraded in a miniature pool of acid, then returned to the surface of the macrophage to be presented to a T-cell. From our point of view, this sequence of events has the crucial consequence that the antigen is radically altered in structure; what the T-cell recognizes may have little resemblance to the original antigen.

In 1986 Øle Werdelin of the University of Copenhagen proposed a unifying hypothesis that the HLA molecules inside the macrophage control the degradation of protein antigens and protect them from extinction. To retain the capacity to stimulate T-cells, the degradation ceases when the antigen has been reduced to short peptide chains with about eight amino acids and bound to an HLA molecule.

It is difficult to provide an up-to-date diagram of what happens within a macrophage because, even as I write, concepts are changing rapidly as new knowledge becomes available. Figure 21 shows that most phagocytic cells have two principal mechanisms. First, extracellular proteins (antigens) are seen approaching from the left. After they have entered the cell, they are first degraded in an acid pool and are then processed by class II HLA molecules. Second, internal proteins formed within cells (including the ones derived from viruses) are processed by class I molecules.

These two well-established mechanisms indicate a paradox, for clinicians know that the reactive arthritis which follows bacterial infections is associated with B27, a class I molecule, and not with class II molecules. For this and other reasons, a few years ago it was suggested that

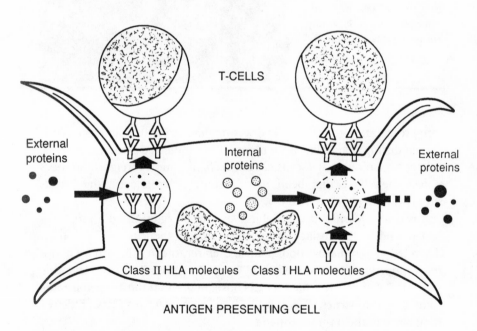

Figure 21 • The processing of proteins in antigen presenting cells, and the presentation of altered protein to lymphocytes.

class I molecules must also have the capacity to handle extracellular proteins (by a third mechanism). In 1990 it was confirmed that there are special cells in which class I as well as class II molecules process external proteins and present them to T-cells, as indicated by the external proteins entering from the right in Figure 21. Then, in 1991, it was proposed that the paradox (and many conflicting results) could be explained by the fact that HLA molecules behave differently in the body than they do when investigated in culture.

Peptides are probably assisted across the cytoplasm by transporter genes that come from the same genetic region as HLA genes. HLA molecules are then created within the cell, apparently forming around peptides. The HLA molecules may transport the peptides to the surface as a constant stream. Alternatively, HLA molecules may rotate to the surface and back, conveying antigen fragments as they go. In this second scheme the ability to present fragments depends on how fast the "conveyor belt" rotates.

As Bjorkman wrote in her letter, these concepts of how HLA molecules dominate antigen presentation emerged as she was completing her work on the three-dimensional structure of these molecules. Moreover, they coincided with a better understanding of T-cell receptor molecules. For the first time, scientists could visualize the all-important interaction of antigen, HLA molecule, and T-cell receptor molecule.

Remembering how Paul Ehrlich was criticized for drawing what he imagined cell receptors might look like, in Figure 22 I have deliberately illustrated my concept of the interaction in a way that can only be imaginary. It is as if the two molecules (HLA and T-cell receptor) can recognize each other by touching fingertips and holding the antigen in both hands, thus allowing a maximum of feedback. On one side of the diagram two other receptors are in physical contact; on the other side, a further receptor intercepts a chemical message.

After so much detail, however interesting, four points deserve special emphasis:

1. The fact that proteins are altered radically during antigen presentation provides the best available explanation of how antigens can provoke inflammation in joints and still escape detection. We have two scenarios. First, the antigens may be engulfed within antigen presenting cells at the site of entry to the body, and altered before entering the

joints; or, second, they may be engulfed and altered immediately upon entering the joints. Whatever happens, clones of T-cells (removed from the synovial fluid or synovium and grown in culture) are now being employed in research to determine exactly what is stimulating them.

2. Although the initial research on antigen processing was conducted on macrophages, other cells—particularly B-cells, dendritic cells, and endothelial cells—can perform the same function.

3. An individual human being has few types of HLA molecules, such as B27 or DR4, and is challenged by an almost infinite number of antigens. Consequently, each type of HLA molecule must be capable of processing thousands of different external and internal proteins and peptides. This means that, despite its beauty, the function of an HLA molecule in processing antigens must be crude, in striking contrast to a T-cell, whose action is specific.

4. The main function of HLA molecules is to protect rather than to damage. The high frequency in the population of HLA genes such as B27 and DR4 must mean that they have strong positive features. Perhaps in

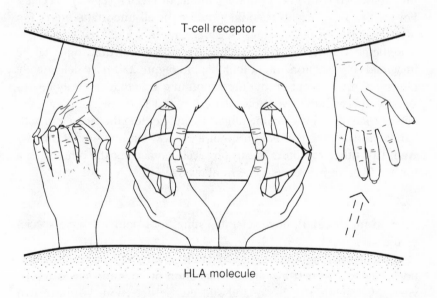

Figure 22 • One concept of the interaction of an antigen, an HLA molecule, and a T-cell receptor.

the past they enabled a distant ancestor, or our parents, to overcome an infection—even tuberculosis or the plague. And perhaps in the present they provide highly desirable characteristics for people who have arthritis. These inherited molecules are not simply defective; they are primarily beneficial.

HLA molecules have another function. So far, we do not know as much about this second function, but it may prove to be at least as important as the first (the involvement of HLA molecules in antigen presentation). The two functions are compatible and operate side by side. This second function could account for several aspects of human disease that we cannot explain solely on the basis of the action of HLA molecules in antigen presentation.

When considering self and nonself, I mentioned Macfarlane Burnet's discovery that the immune system's ability to tolerate self is learned in the embryo. In fact, this is not a once-and-for-all event but a dynamic ongoing process that continues throughout life. We now believe that HLA molecules are active in selecting T-cells, by positive and negative means. The HLA molecules, virtually unique to the individual to whom they belong, can identify T-cells that might attack self and determine that they simply wither away to leave a hole in the T-cell repertoire.

As an example of how this function of HLA molecules might relate to arthritis, consider a person with B27 who has had a salmonella infection and is one hundred times more likely than other people to develop arthritis. What happens could depend on a subtle defect in the way remnants of salmonella are handled by B27 molecules. Or, alternatively, an inadequate response and the development of arthritis could depend on the hole in the T-cell repertoire produced by negative selection.

Techniques for studying clones of T-cells in tissues have become available only recently. Still demanding of time and resources, they have not yet been applied to several important issues in arthritis. For almost twenty years we have been puzzled by the fact that people who have inherited certain HLA molecules show different distributions of joint involvement in arthritis. B27 is particularly related to the spine and to joints in the lower limbs; B8/DR3, to knees, ankles, and wrists; and DR4 and psoriasis, to finger joints. The obvious question is why is this so? Thus far we can only guess the answer. I used to think that the relevant HLA molecules might be more active in certain joints. But we now know that clones of T-cells vary from tissue to tissue, and I prefer the tentative suggestion that the HLA molecules determine the populations of T-cells in individual joints and make them susceptible to arthritis—a possibility that has not yet been tested. A similar argument applies to the fact that people with certain HLA molecules experience the onset of their arthritis at known ages. Could it be that HLA molecules select particular T-cells at particular ages?

Other conundrums interest physicians and might be explained by the T-cell repertoire in individuals. Most people with B27 have no symptoms throughout life. Arthritis is associated with all subtypes of B27—despite the distribution of these subtypes throughout the world. B27 is associated with several diseases, but people with one disease usually do not have any of the other diseases related to B27. The same diseases can occur in the absence of B27, particularly in some populations (such as ankylosing spondylitis in African Americans). Genes for skin and bowel diseases appear to substitute for B27 in conferring susceptibility to arthritis. One attractive possibility is that all of these baffling observations may be caused by the T-cells available, rather than by a defect of the B27 molecules in antigen presentation.

I have long ago indicated that arthritis, and the exciting developments in arthritis research, are complicated. To make these intricate matters easier to understand, let me briefly summarize salient features from the past five chapters.

We all inherit immune systems that are virtually unique. The many components of these systems are primarily beneficial and enable our bodies to recognize, and if necessary eliminate, unwanted proteins and peptides that have entered from the environment or have been formed in our tissues. The immune systems we inherit are not perfect, however, and may make us susceptible to a wide range of different diseases, including arthritis.

We have learned how inherited molecules operate in confronting unwanted peptides, often inside cells of the immune system. Details of these molecules have been established, down to their three-dimensional shape, features of their receptors, and even which four or five amino acids in the molecules recognize, bind, and present peptides to be eliminated. Scientists and physicians in many specialties are captivated by all of these advances. The practical implications for the care of several common diseases are immense.

22

Truth Is Rarely Simple

After examining much of the evidence relating to the causes of arthritis, including the momentous recent discoveries, we need to pause to consider where we are and where we are going.

The only way to understand arthritis is to start by acknowledging that it is complicated; only later is it possible to make it simple. We are faced with many genes, many changes in the host, many environmental triggers, many independent clinical features, and many diseases.

Gregor Mendel turned his back on the flowers in his garden, which were complicated, and concentrated on seeds with individual characteristics, which were simple. Physicians were immediately attracted by Robert Koch's belief that there is an individual microbe for each infectious disease. And all rheumatologists have approved the separation of arthritis into carefully defined, comparatively simple diseases. Although this approach is invaluable, it may also constitute a genuine barrier to understanding and progress, for one of the principal challenges to rheumatology is to explain why each person with arthritis is different.

Ever since the early days of genetics, public interest has centered on inherited characteristics and diseases that follow the simple laws laid down by Mendel—witness the recent debate about the ethics of transferring genes in the treatment of cystic fibrosis and rare inherited disorders such as enzyme defects. In comparison, there has been little public interest in the fact that most heredity results from cooperation among many genes, a cooperation that leads to our own individual characteristics, and sometimes to persistent diseases in hundreds of millions of people. Yet, when we stop to consider the matter, the heredity of complicated characteristics, such as intelligence or the similarity of our facial appearance to that of other family members, cannot be due to one gene. This kind of heredity must be multigenic—from many genes.

The truth is that multigenic heredity determines 80 percent of human characteristics. Genes can aid, block, or enhance one another; and two or more genes, even from different chromosomes, often collaborate in the structure of individual proteins. The heredity of arthritis does not result from a solo by a single gene. Rather, it resembles a symphony by an orchestra of genes and chromosomes playing in harmony—with an occasional discordant note.

Physicians have no difficulty in distinguishing the common, more complex forms of arthritis from diseases that arise from one gene, such as hemophilia, Huntington's chorea, or a specific enzyme defect. On occasion every rheumatologist sees people who have several diseases at the same time, or whose families have several diseases spread among the family members. Doctors often struggle with problems of multigenic heredity.

The reason that this topic had been largely neglected is easy to understand, and I can illustrate from my own experience. After I graduated from medical school, I had no opportunity to apply in clinical practice the information I had learned as a student about multigenic heredity and multifactorial disease. There were no markers that enabled my colleagues and me to study many genes in our patients. Later, though, when we were visiting homes and hospitals in our research project— armed with a battery of relevant genetic markers—we could observe many genes fitting together in families to cause an array of diseases, and then separating again to become less troublesome in subsequent generations. For me personally, HLA molecules made multigenic heredity come to life as an essential part of the diagnosis and care of patients. Since that time, our growing knowledge of multigenic heredity has expanded my initial glimpse into an intricate picture of such dazzling complexity that it is difficult to describe in words.

When people who are familiar with Mendelian genetics learn of a hereditary element in arthritis, they often assume that a fixed number of offspring, like a half or a quarter, will develop a severe form of the condition. In fact, multigenic heredity often causes an identifiable disorder in only a few of those at risk. We have seen that at least 98 percent of people with B27 have no symptoms at any time in their lives; only in families that have arthritis is there a higher frequency of symptoms associated with B27. Also, in multigenic heredity the severity of disease tapers off to nothing in many people. Most individuals who have a given ailment never experience more than trivial symptoms and will probably not be diagnosed. Those who have serious disease are few.

It is understandable that many patients are concerned that if a disorder is inherited, its onset and its progress may be inevitable. They fear that we may be programmed at birth to develop a certain disease, with our individual allocation of the features of that disease due to start at a predestined age, and that nothing can be done without interfering with heredity (which is not advisable). The issue is, fortunately, not that simple. From studies of identical twins we know that even when the genes in two individuals are exactly the same, it is unusual for both of them to develop arthritis. Everything is not preordained by Nature. Twin studies indicate that other factors are even more influential in the causation of arthritis than heredity, age, and gender.

When geneticists investigate our target diseases of ankylosing spondylitis, psoriatic arthritis, and rheumatoid arthritis, they sometimes suggest that the complicated features of arthritis can be explained solely on the basis of the variation in expression of individual genes, as is undoubtedly the case in most diseases caused by a single gene. But this explanation does not fit the known clinical facts about arthritis. For example, several discrete diseases are associated with B27, different clinical features may be seen in family members, and there is an apparent link among nine diseases (two in the intestines, one in the skin, one in the spine, four in the peripheral joints, and one in the eyes). Arthritis is very complicated and must result from multigenic heredity.

The accepted classifications and definitions of the many types of arthritis are essential in diagnosis, treatment, and epidemiology, but that does not prove that there are separate causes for each disorder. My own interpretation of the clinical evidence is that several familiar and carefully defined forms of arthritis probably all arise from basic mechanisms that they share.

The strong influence of HLA molecules in ankylosing spondylitis, reactive arthritis, and psoriatic arthritis allows us to speculate that this group of diseases is predominantly related to the type of cellular response championed by Elie Metchnikoff and James Murphy. In this response HLA molecules and T-cell receptor molecules are especially important. At the other end of the scale, systemic lupus erythematosus is associated with an excess of autoantibodies, but less directly with HLA; so we can suggest that this disease is predominantly related to the type of humoral response championed by Paul Ehrlich, in which antibodies and B-cells are crucial. Between these two extremes we have rheumatoid arthritis, which is associated with both HLA and autoantibodies. Thus, we can surmise that when rheumatoid arthritis is severe, HLA molecules, T-cell receptor molecules, and antibodies all have significant roles.

This perspective enables us to speculate that diverse, nonspecific environmental triggers could initiate and aggravate mild inflammation in anyone's joints. Genes and other host factors would then determine whether this mild inflammation progresses to clinical arthritis, whether it persists as chronic arthritis, and whether the process is diagnosed as ankylosing spondylitis, reactive arthritis, psoriatic arthritis, SLE, or rheumatoid arthritis.

We know for certain that some diseases, such as acute anterior uveitis, psoriasis, ulcerative colitis, and Crohn's disease, are associated with ankylosing spondylitis because of genetic links. In a similar way, scarring of the lungs, dry eyes, and dry mouth appear to have genetic links with rheumatoid arthritis. So it is not difficult to believe that other clinical features and apparent complications of arthritis are also genetically determined. As with the distribution of joints affected and the age of onset, I expect that the T-cell repertoire will account for most unexplained clinical connections.

Knowing that HLA molecules, T-cell receptor molecules, and B-cell receptor molecules work together closely in immune responses, and in different types of arthritis, can we construct a model based on the genetics of these three related molecules that might explain the heredity of susceptibility to our target diseases? The fact that these molecules share structural features proves that they must have had a common ancient origin, early in evolution. They also have an affinity for one another that is probably important in their cooperation in immune responses.

The genetics of these three molecules is critical. The genes for an HLA molecule are on the sixth chromosome; the genes for a T-cell receptor molecule are on the second, seventh, and fourteenth chromosomes; and the genes for a B-cell receptor molecule (an antibody) are on the second, fourteenth, and twenty-second chromosomes. Despite their location on five different chromosomes, it is agreed that the genes for HLA, T-cell receptors, and antibodies are members of the same genetic superfamily.

That is not all, however. Two other inherited factors have not yet been considered. In 1888 it was observed that the blood serum of normal animals contains a substance that is toxic for some microbes. This finding generated considerable interest; and the following year this component of the immune system was called "alexin"—the protective substance. It was Ehrlich who later gave it the appropriate name "complement." The complement system consists of more than twenty proteins. When even one molecule of the first complement is stimulated, a chain reaction triggers rapid multiplication. As a result, the complement response is quick and effective.

Complement can assist the body's defenses in several ways. In the simple example of invasion by bacteria, complement can increase the permeability of small blood vessels so that helpful proteins can reach the site; it can attract polymorphs; it can inflict fatal damage by direct attack on bacteria; or it can coat the bacteria so that they readily adhere to polymorphs or macrophages. The reason for mentioning complement at this stage is that it has a sophisticated genetic system on the sixth chromosome—within the genetic complex that controls HLA molecules. Although complement and HLA have separate functions, it is interesting that both are fundamental in the body's inflammatory responses, and that their genetic systems are linked in the same area of the sixth chromosome. Also, complement is often depleted when SLE is active; we now know that there is a link between the heredity of complement and this disease.

The other inherited factor was discovered in 1955, when it was demonstrated in small animals that skin grafts from males were rejected by females, despite the fact that the males and females were genetically identical except for their sex. This graft rejection was later attributed to the H-Y molecule (which is broadly similar to HLA). The genetic basis for the H-Y molecule is on the sex chromosomes, X and Y. In theory, H-Y (or other genes on the sex chromosomes) could resolve many unexplained aspects of the spectrum of sex ratios in arthritis. However tenuous, this possibility is of immense significance; several million people have arthritic and nonarthritic diseases to which they would have been far less susceptible if they had been of the opposite sex.

The difficulties in assessing this crucial suggestion are obvious. Because we are either male or female, differences of anatomy, hormones, pregnancies, emotions, occupation, environment, and other factors must be taken into account. Hence, we have no evidence so far that the theory is correct, and we have some evidence that it is not. It is far too early, nevertheless, to reject this attractive possibility.

Figure 23 indicates how seven chromosomes might interact in determining susceptibility to arthritis. The genes for HLA and complement are on the same part of the sixth chromosome. The genes for antibodies and for T-cell receptor molecules are on the second, seventh, fourteenth, and twenty-second chromosomes. Also included, solely on theoretical grounds, are the sex chromosomes, X and Y.

We know that from HLA genes alone, many millions of combinations of inherited molecules characterize us as individuals. It has not yet been possible to calculate similar figures for the group of T-cell receptor molecules, but it is probable that their genetics will prove to be even more complex. In a similar way, we already know that the antibody genetic system has the capacity to initiate the production of over 20 billion different antibodies. As if that were not complicated enough, the HLA, T-cell receptor, and antibody genes have a special affinity for one another and are part of the same genetic superfamily. The possible complexity implicit in the interactions among members of this genetic superfamily is incredible—but not beyond human ingenuity.

The Human Genome Project, a massive program involving extensive

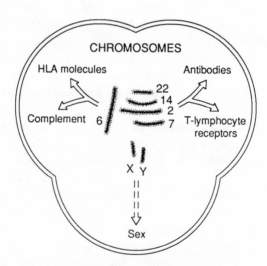

Figure 23 • A schematic drawing that shows how at least seven chromosomes might cooperate in determining susceptibility to arthritis.

international collaboration, is currently determining the sequences of DNA in all of the fifty thousand genes (3 billion nucleotides) on the chromosomes of the human genome. Subject to the availability of funding, within a decade or more computers will be establishing which proteins these genes initiate, and how the genes in the genome produce such an intricate network of proteins. Although it is virtually impossible to comprehend what the results will mean, few will follow the program with more passionate interest than those studying the multigenic heredity of susceptibility to arthritis.

To remind us of the importance of other host factors, we require only a brief summary. Age and sex have a profound influence on when a disease begins and what type of arthritis it is. In some diseases sex hormones probably are important, and in others they are not. I believe that the age when key cells and products of specific genes on sex chromosomes become effective may also be of critical significance.

Malnutrition may be more important than was formerly imagined, especially in parts of the world with marked deprivation. Plans are under way to study the role of chronic malnutrition in susceptibility to arthritis. So far, however, on a broad scale we have only the evidence of selenium deficiency (although far more is known about the part played by malnutrition in bone disease). From clinical work, we know that scurvy, due to vitamin C deficiency, may affect the joints and be difficult to diagnose.

We are learning rapidly about the ways foreign substances enter the body, are transported in the bloodstream, and then enter the joints. We do not know whether the mechanisms vary from individual to individual, making some people unexpectedly susceptible to disease.

Sex hormones almost certainly influence susceptibility to generalized osteoarthritis and to systemic lupus erythematosus. They may also contribute to the causation of rheumatoid arthritis. But we do not yet know how seriously sex hormones influence the remarkable variation in sex ratios in the incidence of other common arthritic diseases.

Pregnancy has a marked effect in ameliorating established rheumatoid arthritis in most women. In addition, the likelihood of developing rheumatoid arthritis may be reduced by repeated pregnancies—or increased by slightly diminished fertility.

Of all these host factors, the most promising advances are being made in studying the critical roles of the emotions, nerves, and adrenal hormones in joint disease. More than any other, this subject may lead to major improvements in the understanding and treatment of arthritis.

One of the principal advantages of understanding the roles of genes and the immune system in arthritis is that it allows us to look afresh at the significance of environmental triggers. With regard to epidemiology, there is little to be gained from extending studies of the type that were so helpful originally. The need now is to concentrate mainly, but not exclusively, on environmental causes, which means that we must be clear about which hypotheses are most suitable to test.

In my opinion, there are now three possible explanations for our principal target diseases—ankylosing spondylitis, psoriatic arthritis, and rheumatoid arthritis—and no hypothesis can be abandoned at this point. The first possibility is that Koch was right, that everywhere in the world there is a specific microbe that causes arthritis and it has escaped detection for a hundred years. The second possibility is that no environmental triggers are involved, that arthritis occurs spontaneously, without external provocation. The third possibility, which I prefer, is that all of the host factors—including heredity, age, gender, hormones, nerves, stress, emotions, and nutrition—determine the clinical details and thus leave environmental triggers with a purely nonspecific role. The initiation and perpetuation of the disease would then depend on many dissimilar common agents, probably varying in different individuals, in different types of arthritis, in different circumstances, and in different parts of the world.

In acute arthritis, and possibly in acute anterior uveitis, one type of microbe alone may be sufficient to cause disease, probably by abrupt mechanisms that differ radically from those in chronic disorders.

If we assume that the role of relevant environmental triggers is nonspecific, we can divide them into two categories: microorganisms and other substances. We agreed earlier that a wide range of live organisms, including bacteria, viruses, and parasites, can enter the joints and induce inflammation of varying degrees of intensity. Prime examples are tuberculosis and Lyme disease. Then there is reactive arthritis, apparently caused by fragments of dead organisms. Examples are arthritis following sexually acquired infection with chlamydia or following dysentery due to salmonella or other organisms. Some arthritis associated with AIDS and schistosomiasis is probably similar. At present it is difficult to categorize either rheumatic fever or erythema nodosum, because less work has been done on synovial tissue in those conditions.

Apart from live microbes and their dead remnants, we are left with other issues that have not been settled. The question of focal sepsis in various parts of the body such as the teeth, sinuses, throat, and lungs has not been studied adequately; it was abandoned upon realizing, with embarrassment, how much unnecessary surgery was being performed. In reviewing this subject, we have no doubt, for instance, that carious teeth result in repeated release of live bacteria into the bloodstream, or that chronic lung infection is associated with autoantibodies in some people and arthritis in others. Our predecessors may have been correct in suggesting that this type of persistent infection is highly relevant.

We certainly have a strong case for conducting surveys of the world's water supplies to find factors that might cause arthritis. We also need to know more about the effects of repeated infections, especially those experienced in childhood, on susceptibility and resistance to arthritis in adult life.

Throughout this book we have encountered chemicals that appear to contribute to inflammatory arthritis. The most persuasive example is the forty-year survey of granite workers in Finland, which revealed a correlation between classic rheumatoid arthritis and prolonged exposure to silica. Moreover, pollution of the air with silica, vinyl chloride, or organic solvents undoubtedly can cause the arthritis associated with systemic sclerosis. Apart from this occupational exposure, however, we are uncertain of the significance of general air pollution in the causation of the common types of arthritis. For those who believe that arthritis became more frequent at the beginning of the nineteenth century and is now becoming less prevalent in developed countries, there is added incentive to study the Industrial Revolution and air pollution at that time. These trends are debatable, though, and recent evidence of the influence of air pollution is confined to one study that showed an increased frequency of rheumatoid factor in industrial towns. Even so, the possibility that air pollution may contribute to arthritis, first confronted in smoke-ridden northern England forty years ago, should be investigated in modern cities, including Los Angeles, that are beleaguered by smog.

The probable contribution of tobacco to the causation and aggravation of rheumatoid arthritis is intriguing. Smoking, both active and passive, causes persistent infection of the sinuses, throat, ears, and lungs.

Also, tobacco remnants spread throughout the body, as witnessed by the effect of nicotine on the brain and the influence of other chemicals on fetal growth. We know that tobacco alters the inner lining of the lungs so other large proteins can enter the circulation, and that many of the clinical conditions associated with tobacco are disorders of small blood vessels. Despite the multitudinous articles reporting the links between tobacco and diseases, many of them fatal, until recently there were no investigations of arthritis. We have solid evidence now that smoking leads to excess rheumatoid factor and other autoantibodies, and controversial evidence that smoking increases the frequency and severity of rheumatoid arthritis. As things stand, one could either conclude that tobacco is irrelevant or speculate that smoking almost doubles the frequency and the severity of rheumatoid arthritis. In light of the fifty million people in the world who have rheumatoid arthritis, relentless pursuit of a reliable answer is mandatory.

Until the recent impressive evidence on the influence of a vegetarian diet, which must now be repeated, no one knew whether diet had any effect on the likelihood of developing arthritis, or on the course of the arthritis once it was established. In spite of strenuous efforts, the subject is well nigh impossible to investigate satisfactorily. As a consequence, people have gone to great lengths and spent vast sums to follow diets that may not help them at all. The entire topic still requires far more research.

There is no doubt that certain drugs lead to systemic sclerosis or to systemic lupus erythematosus. Also, some adverse responses to drugs have been linked to specific HLA molecules or to different genetic markers.

As in a detective story, so in science: when the offenders in the causation of a group of diseases are numerous, it is necessary to investigate all the factors involved until a less complicated solution emerges. At last we can see the simpler theme on which to base new strategies in the prevention and treatment of arthritis.

23

Prospects for Prevention and Treatment

The recent major advances in understanding the scientific aspects of arthritis give us every reason to hope that before long similar advances in prevention and treatment will occur. That time has not yet arrived, however; so I conclude our encouraging story by reviewing what is known about prevention and treatment, and speculating on what may happen in the near future.

In this book I have adopted a broad approach in outlining what has been achieved in research and what remains to be done. Other investigators will, I expect, recognize missing pieces of the jigsaw puzzle that are face up on the table and fit them into the remaining spaces. Only then will prevention and treatment be firmly based on full knowledge of the causes of these diseases. Shortly after the germ theory was shown to be correct, Pasteur reflected, "If the cause of a phenomenon is unknown, all things are hidden, obscure and debatable, but, if the cause is known, everything is clear."

In some respects, our present understanding of many disorders resembles the situation just before there was proof that germs cause disease. No one knew what benefits would result if the hypothesis were correct. Nobody could predict that this knowledge would lead to a host of preventive measures and treatments. But soon everyone understood that clothes belonging to patients dying of cholera must not be washed in the drinking water supply, that typhus was not caused solely by overcrowding, and that disease could be transmitted by insects.

What happened then is common knowledge today and in hindsight seems inevitable. Preventive measures could be targeted accurately. Vaccination against rabies, antitoxin for diphtheria, and Salvarsan for syphilis were quickly introduced—to be followed much later by sulfonamides, penicillin, streptomycin, vaccination against many diseases, and numerous modern treatments. In developed countries the mortality due to infection fell dramatically, and life expectancy increased by more than thirty years. The status of arthritis in the 1990s is similar to that of infection in 1875: soon, one hopes, the causes will be established; the benefits will be immense.

To begin with the crucial subject of disease prevention, I remember with admiration a middle-aged woman whose life had been devastated by years of aggressive rheumatoid arthritis. When, in response to her inquiries, I explained the research we were doing, she said simply, "Well, doctor, I know it is too late to help me; but the thought that you might be able to prevent it happening to other young people makes it all so much easier to bear." She may be correct in assuming that prevention of arthritis will prove easier than its cure.

The first—and immensely controversial—question is whether we can alter the host's susceptibility to arthritis by modifying heredity. The ethical issues that surround multigenic heredity are thorny and should become the subject of widespread, informed debate. Some new issues are involved that cause me deep concern; I am certain that discussion about them should not be restricted to doctors. Remember, we are not considering rare diseases caused by single genes, but common and debilitating diseases associated with the presence of several genes. Arthritis in many millions of people happens to be the best example of this type of multigenic heredity.

At present, by combining clinical examination, reliable history of diseases in the family, and assessment of the available genetic markers, we sometimes can predict (with uncomfortable accuracy) the likelihood and the age of onset of a painful, disabling disease. The problem for the future is that we are powerless to prevent the advances of science, regardless of what the consequences may be. Before long, when we know more about the genetics of HLA, T-cell receptors, and antibodies; when scientists have determined the sequences and interactions of all the genes in the human genome; when disease prediction is more accurate, will we really want to be told what is in store for us many years hence? Having worked in this field for years, I am appalled by the thought that it may become possible to study the blood of an embryo or a newborn infant and forecast that he or she will develop a serious illness at a specific age in adult life.

So far, HLA-B27 is the only inherited molecule that leads to joint disease with enough frequency to justify any consideration of intervention, and then only when arthritis is known to have occurred in close relatives. On occasion, a parent with B27 and arthritis asks me to see his or her child, a few days old, to determine whether the child is likely to develop arthritis as an adult. As a matter of policy, I advise against attempting to predict the future. The truth is that we could determine, in the uterus or after birth, whether the child has HLA-B27. In accordance with Mendel's laws, if one parent has B27 there is an even chance that the child will have B27. In the absence of effective disease prevention, all I could achieve would be to remove the anxiety on the one hand or to intensify it grievously for twenty years or more on the other.

Less frequently, both parents have diseases that are genetically associated, such as spondylitis in one parent and spondylitis, uveitis, or psoriasis in the other parent. They want to determine whether it is wise to have children, and almost invariably this is a difficult problem.

In these two situations there is at most a 50-50 chance of the child's having symptoms in adult life and a much smaller chance of the child's having *troublesome* disease at some time in his or her life. In my experience, none of the parents with disease has wished they had not been born—and I have never advised birth control, and certainly not abortion, solely on the grounds that the child might develop arthritis.

The theoretical possibility of deleting B27 in the process of artificial insemination is something that has not yet been discussed officially. Assume that the father has ankylosing spondylitis and B27. It should be possible to remove ova from the mother, fertilize them artificially, then reinsert only the fertilized ova that do not contain B27. Although I personally would not advocate such a procedure, it warrants earnest ethical deliberation.

In my opinion, attempts to remove B27 in any other way are currently out of the question. It is essential to remember that all HLA molecules, including B27, are primarily beneficial.

A different issue is whether, once we have truly effective preventive measures, we should identify people at risk of developing arthritis. We know that a small proportion of people with B27 develop arthritis following infection with certain bacteria. If that list were extended—and we knew for certain that individuals born with B27, DR4, or B8 are more likely to develop arthritis after, say, air pollution, smoking tobacco, exposure to occupational hazards, or contamination of the water supply—it would theoretically be possible to identify at birth those most at risk and advise them what preventive measures they should take. In a similar category are people with elevated levels of uric acid or rheumatoid factor in the blood months or years before they develop clinical evidence of gout or rheumatoid arthritis.

With regard to other host factors, several additional modes of disease prevention could be used effectively when sufficient research has been done. It is certainly feasible that counseling and other means of diminishing emotional and physical stress could prevent the onset of arthritis, especially in people known to be at risk of developing rheumatoid arthritis. A more realistic approach would be to take measures of this type in the first few months after the onset of symptoms in an attempt to prevent the disease from becoming established.

Apart from selenium deficiency in restricted areas, we do not yet know enough about the influence of malnutrition on arthritis, but it is conceivable that measures to reduce malnutrition could induce resistance to arthritis in millions of people. We already know that weight reduction can prevent osteoarthritis. We cannot yet be sure whether modification of sex-hormone levels can prevent the onset of rheumatoid arthritis; but the prospects are better that this therapy could reduce the severity and progress of the disease.

Next, we should reevaluate the outlook for disease prevention in arthritis by modifying our approach to hygiene and the environment. We cannot avoid wondering why black people in Africa have more frequent and more severe rheumatoid arthritis in towns than in the bush, and whether rheumatoid arthritis is really a recent disease that is now becoming less frequent. Somewhere in those observations lie the clues to how we ought to proceed.

Many general health-care measures are aimed at preventing infections that either kill people or cause infectious diseases; there is far less official interest in mild infections that may cause reactive arthritis a few weeks later. Nor is there major concern about the possibility that the transmission of dead organisms may lead to arthritis. As a minor example of these issues, rheumatologists are concerned by the patients they see with reactive arthritis following salmonella infection. By comparison, the authorities responsible for preventive measures are guided mainly by the incidence of severe diarrhea and death. The result is that endemic salmonella infection in chicken sold in shops continues, based on the expectation that salmonella bacteria are killed during cooking. I do not mean to give the impression that the consequent consumption of the products of dead bacteria plays a role in arthritis; I simply wish to point out that research on this possibility is overdue.

A positive approach to arthritis prevention is seen in the publicity given to the avoidance of tick bites in attempts to prevent Lyme disease. In a similar way, the encouragement to use condoms to prevent AIDS may secondarily reduce the incidence of sexually acquired reactive arthritis. In theory, massive reduction in the frequency and severity of arthritis could result from improved control of parasites, water supply, and focal sepsis. Each is extremely important and deserves extensive research.

Among the nonmicrobial environmental triggers, the most impressive evidence relates to silica, vinyl chloride, organic solvents, and certain drugs in systemic sclerosis; to drugs and other agents in systemic lupus erythematosus; and to silica in rheumatoid arthritis. In each instance, appropriate action has reduced these hazards.

So far we do not have sufficient evidence to advise governments and health authorities on the relevance of air pollution or tobacco to causation of arthritis, but further research might prove that either has profound effects. Similarly, we cannot discard the possibility that painstaking research might identify crucial elements in our diets.

Finally, let us consider drug therapy in the management of arthritis, starting with a brief look at what has been achieved in recent years.

No one who has witnessed the ravages of infection of bones and joints by tubercle bacilli, staphylococci, and other organisms can fail to doubt the transformation that has taken place in the past half-century. The introduction of antibiotics and other effective drugs has brought changes that seemed impossible fifty years ago—and the improvement continues. As one illustration, penicillin has played a significant part in the partial conquest of rheumatic fever.

Cortisone and allied derivatives also have produced miracles in treatment. Polymyalgia rheumatica, a common disease, is now a delight to treat because it disappears within hours of starting cortisone therapy. Nonsteroidal anti-inflammatory drugs bring relief to millions: when given to people with ankylosing spondylitis, these drugs often provide even more remarkable improvement—almost as if their action were specific. In the treatment of gout, we have drugs that block the formation of excess uric acid and thus make this condition one of the most treatable arthritic diseases.

All of this progress is not enough. For most diseases, we can only allow the inflammation to smolder partially checked and modify it to a limited extent. As a consequence, patients, physicians, research workers, and scientists in the pharmaceutical industry are well aware that radical new ideas are required. Fortunately, vast facilities and financial resources are available to develop fresh initiatives.

In the future, the consequences of our much improved understanding of arthritis need not be complicated. A change of emphasis may be all we need. In rheumatoid arthritis, for instance, we have learned that there is an opportunity to reverse the disease during the first year and thereby prevent it from becoming established; that is when the most effective treatments should be given. In theory, prednisone can diminish the production of adhesion molecules by the endothelium in the synovium, reduce the local inflammation, and prevent irreparable damage to small vessels that may lead to persistent arthritis.

Since the recent work on HLA molecules, T-cell receptor molecules, and peptides, various proposals have been made for preventing inflammation by blocking their interaction. One method would be to manufacture synthetic peptides that bind to specific HLA molecules and effectively inactivate them, thereby preventing inflammation rather than interfering with the inflammatory processes after they are in progress. Another approach would be to delete T-cells known to contribute to individual diseases, thereby blocking harmful responses by T-cells.

More fundamental, and more appealing, is the alternative of intercepting foreign antigens before they reach the joint tissues. This might be done at the sites of entry to the body, or as the antigens are being transported in the bloodstream.

The brightest prospect is that of preventing the passage of antigens in the synovial vessels from the bloodstream into the synovial tissues. Several research groups are concentrating on how the linings of the small blood vessels function in the joints, aiming to devise new strategies to prevent the entrance of antigens into the joint tissues, for instance by reducing the production by endothelial cells of molecules that promote the adhesion or migration of white blood cells. All these projects are experimental and, apart from prednisone, such drugs are not yet available for use in treatment. Nevertheless, there is every reason to anticipate major improvements in drug therapy before long.

No one can foresee what other advances in prevention and treatment will ensue. When I first returned to the Royal National Orthopaedic Hospital as a consultant physician, one of my duties was to share in the care of people severely paralyzed by poliomyelitis. Each summer we would admit up to a hundred children and young adults with that appalling condition. While treating those courageous victims, I attended an international conference on poliomyelitis in Madrid, where I learned how much worse the disease could be in other countries. No one mentioned prevention. Shortly afterward, vaccination against poliomyelitis became widely available; as a result, this type of paralysis virtually disappeared from countries with the facilities to mount effective immunization campaigns. With arthritis, there are likely to be many new techniques of prevention and treatment, rather than a single technique such as vaccination. Yet the goal of abolishing the disease is exactly the same.

Looking back to my favorites, Jane and Philip, the question they most wanted answered was, *"When* will doctors know how to prevent or cure arthritis?" They are not alone: all of us have pain at times; a third of the population endure sufficient symptoms to make them believe they have joint problems; over one hundred million adults and children suffer pain and disability due to arthritis. It is a question we cannot ignore.

Further progress requires a widespread appreciation of how much has been learned and how rapidly science has advanced. Arthritis cannot be defeated until the goal is recognized as achievable. When support rises and demand for a cure intensifies, resources for research will multiply. Then arthritis will be conquered—within a few years.

Some Common Disorders

Glossary

Sources and Suggested Readings

Voluntary Health Organizations

Acknowledgments

Index

Some Common Disorders

Ankylosing spondylitis   This is primarily a disease of young adults, with an onset usually between the ages of eighteen and thirty-five. It is more common, and often more severe, in men than in women. "Spondylitis" means inflammation of the spine. "Ankylosing" means becoming rigid, and therefore applies only to the more severe forms of the disease. Many people with this disease have mild symptoms and go through life without a diagnosis of their spinal discomfort. Onset is usually gradual, and the symptoms are often worse in the morning than at other times of day. In addition to lumbar pain, there may be pain between the shoulder blades, in the neck, around the chest, or in the thighs.

Backache   Everyone has backache occasionally, for only a few days at a time. Most people do not consult a physician; they have a hot bath, rest in bed, and take obvious precautions to protect their back from strain or twisting movements. Problems arise only when the pain is particularly severe, when there are additional clinical features (such as sciatica), or when the pain is persistent. In these circumstances it is wise to consult a primary-care physician. When the pain persists for, say, three months, the physician has a difficult task in deciding not only why the pain started, but also why it lasted longer than expected. The possible reasons are numerous and include the personality of the patient, and social and psychological factors, as well as the nature of the physical disorder. It is very rare for there to be a serious cause, such as cancer.

Brachial neuralgia   Sudden, severe pain in the neck and arm due to pressure on one of the nerve roots in the neck is surprisingly common, and occurs in at least one person in twenty between the ages of thirty and sixty years. The cause is not serious and the prognosis is favorable, but many people have pain so severe that they fear cancer. The pain often radiates from the neck to the shoulder and elbow and sometimes to the hand, where there may also be tingling in the fingers. The pain usually begins to subside after ten to fourteen days, and is much improved after four to six weeks.

Depression   Psychological depression is a common factor that aggravates and prolongs relatively minor physical ailments. Most people with depression are reluctant or unwilling to recognize that the condition exists or that it contributes to their symptoms. In such circumstances a physician may temporarily treat the physical disorder to avoid confrontation, and as a means of achieving acceptance of the true diagnosis. Ultimate success in therapy depends on opportunities to ventilate the real issues (sometimes supplemented by antidepressant drugs), rather than on retreat into prolonged and ineffective treatment of the minor physical disorder.

Fibromyalgia   Otherwise healthy people commonly experience ill-defined, widespread, mild to moderate pain, with multiple points of local tenderness and sleep disturbance. Often these symptoms are associated with emotional stress, depression, or a variety of other psychological or social factors. Many factors may cause such symptoms to persist, become acute, and lead to a medical consultation at which a diagnosis of fibromyalgia may be made. This condition sometimes is so severe that it dominates the lives of those who suffer it. Some physicians believe that the best treatment is to identify the underlying social and psychological factors and to seek to help in their resolution; other physicians maintain that there is a physical basis for the disorder and that it should be treated accordingly.

Gout   The principal feature of gout is an attack, or periodically repeated attacks, of severe arthritis, usually confined to a single joint. Often the site is the large joint of the big toe, but it may be elsewhere in the foot or ankle, in a knee, or in the wrist or hand. Without a clear history of such attacks, the diagnosis of gout is seldom made. There is a partial association between clinical gout and raised levels of uric acid (urate) detected by blood tests. Attacks of gout seldom occur with normal blood tests, but most people with increased uric acid do not have gout, even when they have joint symptoms. Gout is rare in women under the age of fifty. In recent years drug therapy (especially for high blood pressure) has often had the side effect of increasing the body's uric acid and inducing clinical gout—in women almost as much as in men. The long-term treatment is highly successful—usually by pills that markedly reduce the body's production of urate.

Heberden's nodes   Women over the age of forty frequently develop small nodules, known as Heberden's nodes, near the end joints of their fingers. Men may develop similar nodes, usually as the result of former injuries to their fingers. Severe pain in this condition is rare. When patients consult their physicians, it is generally because of concern about the appearance of the nodes or because of understandable, but unjustified, fear of impending arthritis.

Lyme disease   Tick bites may result in an infection that leads to a characteristic illness with arthritis, rash, and other clinical features. This disease has caused considerable concern in areas such as New England, where it occurs with unusual frequency. In recent years Lyme disease has been the subject of much publicity and extensive research.

Myalgic encephalomyelitis (ME), also known as postviral syndrome
By definition, ME follows an acute viral infection; it is characterized by disabling fatigue, widespread discomfort, sleep disturbance, and unusual forms of depression. Many physicians are keeping an open mind about whether this is primarily a psychological disorder or whether there is a physical element to the condition. The evidence for a physical cause is incomplete.

Osteoarthritis   The term "osteoarthritis" is misleading, for it implies that the condition is primarily a form of inflammation of the joints, which is not true. Instead, osteoarthritis is mainly a process of mechanical joint failure, the final common pathway of many disorders. In joint failure the cartilage and underlying bone become worn, leading to local tissue damage and attempts at tissue repair. All of our joints begin to wear from the age of twenty on, so that by age fifty most of us have changes in our joints due to osteoarthritis that are visible on x-ray.

Osteoporosis   In this condition the chemical composition of the bones is normal, but the substance of the bone is markedly diminished, making the bones weak and liable to fracture. After adolescence all of us gradually lose bone substance, decade after decade, and it is inevitable that by old age our bones will be thin and weak. In some people, particularly in women, this loss of bone occurs more rapidly than in others, and there is an acceleration of bone loss at the time of the female menopause. Osteoporosis also results from other diseases, particularly arthritis, and from prolonged treatment with cortisone-like drugs. The symptoms of osteoporosis are mostly confined to the spine and hips. In the spine, collapse of a vertebra (usually above the waist) may cause sudden, severe pain, usually in an older person. In the hips, fractures due to osteoporosis are common in elderly women. When osteoporosis is severe in the limbs, as when it is secondary to arthritis, spontaneous fracture of other limb bones may occur.

Polymyalgia rheumatica   A condition of elderly people, polymyalgia rheumatica is characterized by stiffness and discomfort, particularly of the shoulders, hips, neck, and lumbar region. The onset is often insidious, with only a diffuse sense of stiffness—little more than is suffered by most people. Symptoms gradually become more severe over a period of weeks or months. Response to treatment with cortisone-like drugs is excellent.

Psoriatic arthritis   This distinct form of arthritis is usually associated with the common skin disorder psoriasis. The main characteristic of psoriatic arthritis is the distribution of joints involved. As in rheumatoid arthritis, there is usually finger arthritis; and as in ankylosing spondylitis, there is often inflammation of joints in the spine. Unlike rheumatoid arthritis, psoriatic arthritis is not associated with rheumatoid factor in the blood.

Reactive arthritis   This is an inflammation in one or more joints (in which no live organisms are found) as a delayed reaction to infection elsewhere in the body. Symptoms of the arthritis usually begin two to four weeks after the initial infection and subside over the next three months. Two types of reactive arthritis are commonly recognized: the first occurs predominantly in men and follows sexually transmitted infection; the second occurs equally in both sexes and follows dysentery.

Rheumatoid arthritis   The most important and most damaging of all types of arthritis, rheumatoid is also the most mysterious. It occurs in approximately 1 percent of the population in all but a few countries of the world. The commonest onset is with slowly progressive pain and swelling in the finger joints of middle-aged women. But arthritis may begin in any joint, with presenting symptoms that are highly variable. Fatigue, weight loss, and anemia are common. A protein called rheumatoid factor is found in the blood of most people with rheumatoid arthritis.

Sciatica   Sciatica is characterized by pain in the leg due to pressure on a nerve root in the lumbar region. In young adults the cause is usually a disc protrusion; in older people, it may be osteoarthritis. Each nerve root gives rise to a characteristic distribution of pain, numbness, and tingling in the leg and foot. Examination may disclose areas of numbness and local weakness, or diminished nerve reflexes.

Systemic lupus erythematosus (SLE)   This disorder occurs mainly in women younger than forty years of age; often it begins or is aggravated during or soon after pregnancy. It is a general illness of which arthritis is only one part. Skin, kidneys, lungs, heart, eyes, or brain may be affected. Joints and tendons are often painful, but the joints are seldom markedly swollen and rarely permanently damaged. Although one of the characteristics of SLE is the presence of autoantibodies in the blood, it has not been established whether these autoantibodies are important components of the inflammation—or simply interesting by-products of the disease process.

Glossary

Acromegaly   A chronic disease characterized by large bones and joints.

Acute anterior uveitis (iritis)   An inflammation of sudden onset inside the front of the eye.

Adrenal glands   Two small endocrine glands located above the kidneys.

Adrenaline (epinephrine)   A hormone secreted by the adrenal medulla.

AIDS   Acquired immunodeficiency syndrome.

Amino acid   A chemical that is a basic unit of protein.

Ankylosing spondylitis   A confusing term that now includes spondylitis, uveitis, and peripheral arthritis, but that originally meant complete rigidity of the spine due to a particular form of inflammation.

Ankylosis   Complete immobility of a joint due to disease of that joint.

Anthrax   A virulent infection characterized by pustules and acquired from animals.

Antibiotic   A substance capable of killing or inhibiting the growth of microbes.

Antibody   A special protein (immunoglobulin) that reacts with an antigen.

Antigen   A substance that can stimulate a specific immune response in which there is a reaction by either antibodies or cells.

Antitoxin   An antibody produced against a toxin.

Arthritis   Inflammation of a joint or joints.

Arthropods   The largest group of invertebrates, including insects, spiders, and crustacea.

Arthroscope   A slim, tubular instrument for looking inside joints.

Atom   The smallest portion of matter with the characteristics of a particular chemical element that can take part in a chemical reaction.

Autoantibody   An antibody directed against one's own tissues.

Autoimmune   Relating to an immune reaction in response to one's own tissues.

Bacteriology   The study of bacteria.

Bacterium   An organism comprising a single cell with an ill-defined nucleus.

B-cell   A lymphocyte involved in the synthesis of antibodies.

Behçet's disease   An uncommon disease involving many body systems, including joints.

Blood vessels   Walled canals through which blood circulates.

Bone   The hard part of the skeleton, made up of dense connective tissue and calcified material.

Brachial neuralgia   Pain in the neck and arm due to pressure on a nerve root.

Calcium pyrophosphate dihydrate   A chemical sometimes deposited in joint cartilage as crystals.

Capillaries   Hair-like blood vessels joining small arteries and small veins.

Capsule   A dense envelope that surrounds a joint or other similar structure.

Cartilage   Tough, semitranslucent, bluish-white, elastic tissue that is usually connected to bone.

Cell   The biological unit from which living organisms and tissues are built.

Chemotherapy   The use of chemical agents in treatment.

Cholera   An epidemic, infectious disease characterized by extremely severe dysentery and vomiting.

Chondrocyte   A cartilage cell.

Chorea   A disease mainly affecting children, characterized by involuntary movements.

Chromosomes   Individual thread-like structures in the cell nucleus, composed of DNA.

Collagen   The major molecule of connective tissue, and the most abundant protein in the body.

Conjunctivitis   Inflammation of the protective covering around the eye.

Connective tissue   Diffuse tissue throughout the body, derived from the mesoderm of the embryo, made up of fibers and an amorphous substance that provide support, and cells (including macrophages, lymphocytes, and polymorphs) that provide defense.

Contagion   Transmission of an infectious disease by physical contact.

Cortisone   A drug related to a hormone secreted by the adrenal cortex.

Crepitation   A crackling sound.

Crohn's disease   A persistent inflammation of the intestine of unknown cause, described by Burrill Crohn.

Crystallography   The study of crystals by x-ray diffraction.

Culture   The technique of growing microbes, cells, tissues, or organs under artificial conditions.

Cystic fibrosis   An inherited disease affecting principally the lungs and the pancreas.

Cytoplasm   The contents of a cell (excluding the nucleus).

Diphtheria   A virulent infection characterized by involvement of the throat and production of a toxin.

Diuretic   A drug that increases the amount of urine.

DNA (deoxyribonucleic acid)   Genetic material.

Dominant   One of a pair of genes that will produce its effect without assistance from its counterpart.

Dysentery   Inflammation of the colon with severe diarrhea.

Endothelial cells   Cells lining hollow parts within the body; used in this book to describe the cells lining blood vessels.

Enzyme   A protein substance that accelerates a biochemical reaction.

Epidemiology   The study of diseases and their characteristics within defined populations.

Episodic arthritis Arthritis that recurs in brief attacks.

Erythema chronicum migrans A slowly enlarging red rash.

Erythema nodosum A disease characterized by round, tender, red swellings in the skin.

Estrogen A substance with the effect of estradiol (a hormone of the ovaries).

Familial Mediterranean fever A disease characterized by acute attacks of severe pain in the joints, abdomen, or chest.

Fermentation A chemical change produced by enzymes widely used in the production of alcoholic beverages.

Fibromyalgia A condition characterized by widespread mild to moderate pain, with multiple points of tenderness.

Filariasis A common infection caused by worms.

Gene One of a series of units arranged along the line of a chromosome.

Genome A complete set of genes and chromosomes.

Germ A microscopic organism.

Gout A disease characterized by attacks of arthritis.

Graft Tissue moved from one site to a different site, in the same or another individual.

Heberden's nodes Firm, bony nodules at the ends of the fingers, associated with osteoarthritis.

Helix A structure with a spiral shape.

Hemoglobin The respiratory pigment in red blood cells.

Hemophilia A severe bleeding disease that affects males and is transmitted by females.

Hepatitis Inflammation of the liver.

Herpes A virus causing inflammation of the skin or genitals with small, deep-seated blisters.

HLA A molecule involved in the recognition of foreign or abnormal substances; the name derives from Human, Leukocyte (white cell), and A (the first such molecule discovered).

Hormone A specific chemical substance; formerly confined to substances made by endocrine glands and secreted into the blood, but now including similar substances which influence neighboring cells or even the cell that makes the hormone.

Host   Any organism, including a human, in which or on which another organism (a microbe) can live as a parasite.

Humor   Any fluid of the body.

Humoral   Concerning a fluid of the body.

Hypertrophic pulmonary osteoarthropathy (HPOA)   A condition of the joints (particularly the knees, ankles, and wrists), usually associated with lung disease.

Hypothalamus   A part of the brain below the thalamus.

Immune system   A collective term for the body's defenses against foreign and abnormal substances.

Immunity   Protection against an infective or allergic disease, or against a toxic substance.

Immunoglobulins   Antibodies and other proteins related to them.

Immunological tolerance   Reduction or elimination of the ability of an individual to react specifically to an antigen.

Immunology   The study of immunity and its phenomena.

Infection   The invasion of the body by microbes and their subsequent multiplication.

Inflammation   Redness, heat, swelling, and pain in response to a variety of abnormal stimuli.

Inoculate   To transfer or implant material containing microbes or their products.

Interleukin   One of a group of substances that stimulate and activate cells.

Joint   A junction between two or more bones.

Kashin-Beck disease   An endemic disease characterized by worn joints, which occurs especially in children.

Lavage   Washing out, or irrigation (in this book applied to the joints).

Life cycle   A series of phases from a particular stage in one generation to the same stage in the next generation.

Ligament   A thickened band of white fibrous tissue that connects bones and provides support.

Lipopolysaccharide   A component of certain bacteria.

Lyme disease   A disease caused by *Borrelia burgdorferi.*

Lymph   The pale-yellow fluid found in lymph vessels.

Lymph gland   An encapsulated collection of lymph tissue in the course of a lymph vessel.

Lymphocyte   A small cell with a prominent, round nucleus, which makes many contributions to an immune response.

Lymph vessel   A fine transparent channel that conveys lymph.

Macrophage   A large cell of critical importance in the immune system.

Matrix   Intercellular tissue.

Meniscus   A semilunar cartilage in the knee.

Microbe   An alternative term for "microorganism"; any living entity of microscopic size.

Microbiology   The study of microorganisms; a broader and more correct term than "bacteriology."

Microorganism   Any living entity of microscopic size.

Molecule   The simplest unit of a chemical compound that can retain its independent existence and its characteristic properties, consisting of two or more atoms held together by chemical bonds.

Multigenic   Involving many genes.

Mumps   A viral disease that includes swelling of the parotid glands.

Mutation   Alteration in a gene.

Myalgic encephalomyelitis (ME)   A condition in which prolonged fatigue and widespread discomfort follow an apparent acute viral infection. Also known as the postviral syndrome.

Myoglobin   A respiratory pigment in muscle cells.

Nerve fibers   The long, thin extensions of nerve cells, typically found as bundles within nerves.

Nervous system   A collective term that includes all the nerves of the body and the brain.

Neuropathic joint   A joint that is severely worn due to disordered function of its nerve supply.

Nonsteroidal   Not like cortisone.

Nucleic acid   An acid that is combined with proteins in a cell, in DNA and RNA.

Nucleotide   A repeating component of nucleic acids that contains a phosphate, a sugar, and an organic base.

Nucleus   The central core of a cell.

Orthopedic   Relating to surgery of the locomotor system.

Osteitis condensans ilii   A condition of the sacroiliac joints, usually following pregnancy or a mechanical strain.

Osteoarthritis   A misleading word that denotes wearing of a joint due to joint failure, while implying—incorrectly—a bony disorder related to inflammation of a joint.

Osteomalacia   Softening of the bones.

Osteomyelitis   Inflammation of bone and bone marrow.

Osteoporosis   Thinning of the bones.

Parasite   An organism that lives on another living organism at the expense of the latter.

Parvovirus   A small DNA virus.

Pathology   Study of the causes of disease and the effects of disease on the structure and function of the body.

Periosteum   Dense connective tissue surrounding those parts of a bone not covered by cartilage.

Peripheral arthritis   Arthritis of joints that are not in the spine.

Phagocyte   A cell that has the capacity to ingest small foreign and abnormal substances, including microorganisms.

Physiology   The study of phenomena in living organisms, and their consequences.

Pituitary   An endocrine gland at the base of the brain.

Plague   An epidemic, often fatal disease caused by *Pasteurella pestis*.

Polymorph   A small, mobile cell with a nucleus that takes many shapes; a polymorphonuclear cell.

Polymyalgia rheumatica   A condition of elderly people characterized by stiffness, particularly of the shoulders.

Polymyositis   Diffuse inflammation of many muscles.

Postviral syndrome   A condition in which prolonged fatigue and widespread discomfort follow an apparent acute viral infection. Also known as myalgic encephalomyelitis, or ME.

Prednisone, prednisolone   Two drugs similar to each other and to cortisone.

Prospective   A term applied to a forward-looking project that records events as they develop.

Protein   A class of complex combinations of amino acids—which are essential components of all living cells, being responsible for growth and maintenance of all tissues.

Protozoa   A subkingdom of unicellular and acellular organisms.

Psoriasis   A patchy, chronic inflammation of the skin.

Psoriatic arthritis   Arthritis associated with psoriasis.

Raynaud's phenomenon   An attack of whiteness, blueness, and redness of the hands and/or feet; named for a Paris physician, Maurice Raynaud.

Reactive arthritis   Arthritis as a reaction to infection, in which no live organisms are found in the joints.

Receptor   A specialized molecule on the surface of a cell that reacts with antigens, hormones, drugs, and other stimuli.

Recessive   A gene that will produce its effect only in combination with its counterpart; the opposite of dominant.

Reflex dystrophy   Reflex changes in the joints and other tissues, usually in response to a source of pain.

Reiter's disease   A widely used name for reactive arthritis.

Reticuloendothelial system   The system of specialized cells throughout the body that ingest foreign particles.

Rheumatic fever   An acute illness, usually in children, that may cause fever, arthritis, and sometimes heart disease.

Rheumatism   An outdated word based on the misconception of the ancient Greeks that illness is caused by the flowing of humors.

Rheumatoid arthritis   A particular type of arthritis of unknown cause.

Rheumatoid factor   An unusual protein associated with rheumatoid arthritis.

Rheumatology   The study of disorders of joints, bones, ligaments, nerves, and muscles; derived from the misconceived word "rheumatism."

Rickettsiae   Microorganisms that resemble bacteria in their size and cell division, and resemble viruses in that they are obliged to live within cells of the host.

RNA (ribonucleic acid)   Genetic material.

Ross River virus   An RNA virus that has caused epidemics of fever and arthritis in Australia and some islands of the Western Pacific.

Rubella   A mild viral disease that causes rash and sometimes arthritis.

Sarcoidosis   A generalized disease of unknown cause involving the reticuloendothelial system.

Scarlet fever   An acute infectious illness caused by streptococci; formerly called scarlatina.

Schistosomiasis   A common disease caused by parasitic flukes.

Sciatica   Pain in the leg due to pressure on a nerve root.

Scleritis   An inflammation of the outer opaque coating of the eye.

Scleroderma   A former name for systemic sclerosis, now largely abandoned.

Selenium   A nonmetallic element similar to sulfur in its chemical properties.

Sequencing   Determining the identity of a series of amino acids in a protein or peptide, or of nucleotides in DNA or RNA.

Sjögren's syndrome   A disorder produced by deficient secretion of the lacrimal, salivary, and other glands.

Smallpox   A generalized acute viral infection, now eradicated.

Spirochete   A member of an order of bacteria characterized by their spiral shape and the long filaments attached to their bodies.

Spondylitis   A diffuse, chronic inflammation of the spine.

Streptomycin   An antibiotic used principally in the treatment of tuberculosis.

Stress   A nonspecific response of the body to any demand.

Sympathetic nerves   Nerves supplying viscera, glands, heart, blood vessels, and special muscles.

Synovial fluid   The fluid in the joint space.

Synovitis   Inflammation of the synovium.

Synovium   The soft, thin lining inside most joints.

Syphilis   A contagious, sexually transmitted disease.

Systemic   Relating to the body as a whole.

Systemic lupus erythematosus (SLE)   A disease of connective tissue, skin, joints, lungs, kidneys, heart, and nervous system.

Systemic sclerosis   A disease that thickens the skin and may involve the heart, lungs, gut, kidneys, or muscles.

T-cell   A lymphocyte involved in cellular immunity.

Tendon   A discrete band of bundles of connective tissue by which muscles are attached to bone.

Tenosynovitis   Inflammation of the synovium that surrounds tendons.

Thoracic duct   A large lymph vessel starting in the abdomen and emptying into a large vein in the neck.

Tick   A blood-sucking insect.

Tissue   The collection of similar cells and intercellular material of which animals and plants are made.

Tissue-typing   A technique for determining the HLA molecules in an individual.

Tobacco mosaic disease   A viral disease of tobacco plants.

Toxin   A poisonous substance produced by certain bacteria.

Transplant   To graft living tissue or an organ from one part of the body to another, or from one person to another.

Trophic   Concerning nutrition.

Trypanosomiasis   A disease caused by a particular type of protozoa and transmitted by insects.

Tsetse fly   The fly that transmits the protozoa of trypanosomiasis from cattle to humans in Africa.

Tuberculosis   A highly variable infectious disease that often involves the lungs but may affect any tissue.

Typhoid   An acute infectious disease characterized by fever, rash, and severe diarrhea.

Typhus   A group of infectious diseases conveyed by the bite of insects inhabited by rickettsiae.

Ulcerative colitis   A persistent inflammation of the intestine of unknown cause.

Urate   A salt of uric acid.

Urethritis   Inflammation of the canal through which urine passes when leaving the bladder.

Uric acid   A normal constituent of the body, present in excess in gout.

Vaccination   Originally the inoculation of the live viruses of cowpox; broadened in meaning by Louis Pasteur to include the use of all organisms, alive or dead, to produce immunity to a particular disease.

Vertebral hyperostosis   A condition in which there is excess bone growth in the spine.

Virus   An organism comprising mainly genetic material, which is small enough to pass through filters that retain bacteria.

Vitamin B$_{12}$ A vitamin used in the treatment of pernicious anemia.

Weil's disease (rat-bite fever)   An infectious disease characterized by liver disease and caused by a particular spirochete.

White blood cell (leukocyte)   Any of the colorless cells of the immune system found in normal blood.

Whooping cough   An infectious disease, particularly in children, characterized by frequent attacks of coughing.

X-ray   An electromagnetic radiation with a short wavelength.

Sources and Suggested Readings

General References

Brewerton, D. A. 1988. Causes of arthritis. *Lancet*, ii: 1063–66.

Nobel Foundation, ed. 1972. *Nobel: The Man and His Prizes*, 3rd ed. New York: American Elsevier Publishing Company.

Root-Bernstein, R. S. 1989. *Discovering*. Cambridge, Massachusetts: Harvard University Press.

1. The Search for Germs

Bouchard, M. 1894. Arthropathies (rhumatisme subaigu chronique); recherches microchiennes experimentale. *La Semaine Medicale*, 11:387.

Brock, T. D. 1961. *Milestones in Microbiology*. London: Prentice-Hall.

Brock, T. D. 1988. *Robert Koch: A Life in Medicine and Bacteriology*. Madison, Wisconsin: Science Tech Publishers.

Dubos, R. 1988. *Pasteur and Modern Science*. Madison, Wisconsin: Science Tech Publishers.

Foster, W. D. 1970. *A History of Medical Bacteriology and Immunology*. London: Heinemann Medical Books.

Mullett, C. F. 1956. *The Bubonic Plague and England*. Lexington: University of Kentucky Press.

Various authors. 1875. Germ theory of disease. *Lancet*, i:409, 444, 501, 511, 514, 573, 619, 682, 709.

2. The Body's Defenses

Ehrlich, P. 1900. On immunity with special reference to cell life. *Proceedings of the Royal Society*, 66: 424–448.

Lowy, I. 1989. James Bumgardner Murphy and the early discovery of the role of lymphocytes in immune reactions. *Bulletin of the History of Medicine*, 63: 356–391.

Malkin, H. M. 1984. Julius Cohnheim (1839–1884): his life and contributions to pathology. *Annals of Clinical and Laboratory Science*, 14:335–342.

Marquardt, M. 1949. *Paul Ehrlich*. London: Heinemann Medical Books.

Maulitz, R. C. 1978. Rudolf Virchow, Julius Cohnheim and the program of pathology. *Bulletin of the History of Medicine*, 52: 162–182.

Metchnikoff, E. 1908. *Immunity in Infectious Diseases*. Cambridge: Cambridge University Press.

Murphy, J. B. 1926. *The Lymphocyte in Resistance to Tissue Grafting, Malignant Disease, and Tuberculous Infection: An Experimental Study*. New York: Rockefeller Institute for Medical Research, monograph no. 21.

Silverstein, A. M. 1989. *A History of Immunology*. San Diego: Academic Press.

4. Bacteria, Alive or Dead

Brock, T. D. 1988. *Robert Koch: A Life in Medicine and Bacteriology*. Madison, Wisconsin: Science Tech Publishers.

Brodie, B. B. 1818. *Pathological and Surgical Observations on Diseases of the Joints*. London: Longman.

Glover, J. A. 1930. The incidence of acute rheumatism. *Lancet*, i: 499–505.

Good, A. E. 1970. Hans Reiter, 1881–1969. *Arthritis and Rheumatism*, 13: 296–297.

Granfors, K., S. Jalkanen, A. A. Lindberg, et al. 1990. Salmonella lipopolysaccharide in synovial cells from patients with reactive arthritis. *Lancet*, 335: 685–688.

Keat, A., J. Dixey, C. Sonnex, et al. 1987. Chlamydia trachomatis and reactive arthritis: the missing link. *Lancet*, i: 72–74.

Paronen, I. 1948. Reiter's disease, a study: 344 cases observed in Finland. *Acta Medica Scandinavica*, 212 (suppl.): 1–112.

Pearson, C. M. 1956. Development of arthritis, periarthritis and periostitis in rats given adjuvant. *Proceedings of the Society of Experimental Biology and Medicine*, 91: 95–101.

Sairanen, E., I. Paronen, and H. Mahonen. 1969. Reiter's syndrome: a follow-up study. *Acta Medica Scandinavica*, 185: 57–63.

Wharton, M. 1983. Sir Benjamin Brodie, Bt. (1783–1862). *Annals of the Royal College of Surgeons of England*, 65: 418–419.

Willan, R. 1808. *Cutaneous Diseases*. London: J. Johnson.

5. Tales of Ticks in America

Beatty, W. K. 1981. Howard Taylor Ricketts—imaginative investigator. *Proceedings of the Institute of Medicine, Chicago*, 34: 46–48.

Steere, A. C., S. E. Malawista, D. R. Snydman, et al. 1977. Lyme arthritis: an epidemic of oligoarticular arthritis in children and adults in three Connecticut communities. *Arthritis and Rheumatism,* 20: 7–17.

6. Access to the Joints

Aschoff, L. 1924. *Lectures of Pathology.* New York: Paul B. Hoeber.

Atkin, S. L., M. Kamel, A. M. A. El-Hady, et al. 1986. Schistosomiasis and inflammatory polyarthritis. *Quarterly Journal of Medicine,* 229: 479–487.

Doury, P., S. Pattin, B. Dienot, et al. 1977. Les rhumatismes parasitaires. *Semaine Hôpital, Paris,* 53: 1359–63.

Florey, H. F. 1970. *General pathology,* 4th ed. London: Lloyd-Luke.

Girges, M. R. 1966. Schistosomal arthritis. *Rheumatism,* 22: 108.

Goodgame, R. W. 1990. AIDS in Uganda—clinical and social features. *New England Journal of Medicine,* 323: 383–389.

Hughes, S. S. 1977. *The Virus: A History of the Concept.* London: Heinemann Medical Books.

Kuhns, J. G., and H. L. Weatherford. 1936. Role of the reticulo-endothelial system in the deposition of colloidal and particulate matter in articular cavities. *Archives of Surgery,* 33: 68–82.

Rowe, I. F., S. M. Forster, M. H. Seifert, et al. 1989. Rheumatological lesions in individuals with human immunodeficiency virus infection. *Quarterly Journal of Medicine,* N.S. 73, no. 272: 1167–84.

Williams, G. 1961. *Virus Hunters.* Rugby, England: Jolly and Barber.

Winchester, R., D. H. Bernstein, H. D. Fischer, et al. 1897. The co-occurrence of Reiter's syndrome and acquired immunodeficiency. *Annals of Internal Medicine,* 106: 19–26.

7. Three Key Diseases

Guillain, G. 1959. *J.-M. Charcot—1825–1893: His Life—His Work,* ed. and trans. P. B. Pearce Bailey. New York: Hoeber.

Landré-Beauvais, A. J. 1985. *Thèse: Doit-on admettre une nouvelle espèce de goutte sous la dénomination de goutte asthénique primitive?* Paris: Editions Louis Pariente.

Porter, R. 1987. *Disease, Medicine and Society in England, 1550–1860.* London: Macmillan.

8. The Many Faces of Arthritis

Behçet, H. 1940. Some observations on the clinical picture of the so-called triple symptom complex. *Dermatologica,* 81: 73–83.

Maricq, H. R., M. N. Johnson, C. L. Whetstone, and E. C. LeRoy. 1976. Capillary abnormalities in polyvinyl chloride production workers. *Journal of the American Medical Association,* 236: 1368–71.

Rodnan, G. P., T. G. Benedek, T. A. Medsger, et al. 1967. The association of progressive systemic sclerosis (scleroderma) with coal-miner's pneumoconiosis and other forms of silicosis. *Annals of Internal Medicine,* 66: 323–334.

Silverstein, A. M. 1989. *A History of Immunology.* San Diego: Academic Press.

Walsh, K. I., and C. M. Black. 1988. Environmental and genetic factors in scleroderma. In *Systemic Sclerosis: Scleroderma,* ed. M. I. V. Jayson and C. M. Black. London: John Wiley.

9. One Gene, One Disease

Dixey, J., A. N. Redington, R. C. Butler, et al. 1988. The arthropathy of cystic fibrosis. *Annals of the Rheumatic Diseases,* 47: 218–223.

Heller, H., E. Sohar, and L. Sherf, 1958. Familial Mediterranean fever. *Archives of Internal Medicine,* 102: 50–71.

Judson, H. R. 1979. *The Eighth Day of Creation: The Makers of the Revolution in Biology.* New York: Simon and Schuster.

Olby, R. 1974. *The Path to the Double Helix.* London: Macmillan.

Olby, R. 1985. *Origins of Mendelism,* 2nd ed. Chicago: University of Chicago Press.

Orel, V. 1984. *Mendel.* Oxford: Oxford University Press.

Perutz, M. 1989. *Is Science Necessary?* London: Barrie and Jenkins.

Sayre, A. 1978. *Rosalind Franklin and DNA.* New York: Norton.

Watson, J. D. 1968. *The Double Helix.* London: Weidenfeld and Nicolson.

10. Joint Failure

Cecil, R. L., and B. H. Archer. 1926. Classification and treatment of chronic arthritis. *Journal of the American Medical Association,* 87: 741–746.

Kellgren, J. H., and E. Moore. 1952. Generalized osteoarthritis and Heberden's nodes. *British Medical Journal,* 1: 181–187.

Marti, B., M. Knobloch, A. Tschopp, et al. 1989. Is excessive running predictive of degenerative hip disease? Controlled study of former elite athletes. *British Medical Journal,* 299: 91–93.

McCarty, D. J., and J. L. Hollander. 1961. Identification of urate crystals in gouty synovial fluid. *Annals of Internal Medicine,* 54: 452–460.

Nesterov, A. I. 1964. The clinical course of Kashin-Beck disease. *Arthritis and Rheumatism,* 7: 29–40.

Waugh, W. 1990. *John Charnley: The Man and the Hip.* London: Springer-Verlag.

Yang, J. 1990. Epidemiological studies on the causes of Kashin-Beck disease.

Proceedings of the International Workshop on Kashin-Beck Disease and Non-communicable Diseases, pp. 63–78. Beijing: Chinese Academy of Preventive Medicine.

11. Age and Sex

Talal, N., ed. 1979. Sex factors, steroid hormones, and the host response. *Arthritis and Rheumatism*, 22: 1153–1313.

12. Other Common Causes of Pain

Brewerton, D. A. 1957. Hand deformities in rheumatoid disease. *Annals of the Rheumatic Diseases*, 16: 183–197.

13. Adrenal Hormones

Bishop, P. M. F. 1955. Dr. Addison and his work. *Guy's Hospital Reports*, 104: 275–294.

Bliss, M. 1982. *The Discovery of Insulin*. Toronto: McClelland and Stewart.

Cannon, W. B. 1932. *The Wisdom of the Body*. London: Kegan Paul, Trench, Trubner.

Hench, P. S., E. C. Kendall, C. H. Slocumb, and H. F. Polley. 1949. The effect of a hormone of the adrenal cortex (17-hydroxy-11-dehydrocortisone: compound E) and of pituitary adrenocorticotrophic hormone on rheumatoid arthritis. *Proceedings of the Staff Meetings of the Mayo Clinic*, 24: 181–197.

Selye, H. 1952. *The Story of the Adaptation Syndrome*. (Told in the form of informal, illustrated lectures.) Montreal: Acta, Inc.

14. The Nervous System

Finsterbush, A., and B. Friedman. 1975. The effect of sensory denervation on rabbits' knee joints. *Journal of Bone and Joint Surgery*, 57-A: 949–956.

Guillain, G. 1959. *J.-M. Charcot—1825–1893: His Life—His Work*, ed. and trans. P. B. Pearce Bailey. New York: Hoeber.

Wolff, H. G. 1961. Man's nervous system and disease. *Archives of Neurology*, 5: 235–243.

16. Populations and Families

Cockburn, W. C., and F. Assaad. 1973. Some observations on the communicable diseases as public health problems. *Bulletin of the World Health Organization*, 49: 1–12.

Greenwood, B. M. 1968. Autoimmune disease and parasitic infections in Nigerians. *Lancet*, ii: 380–382.

Kellgren, J. H. 1966. Joseph J. Bunim memorial lecture: epidemiology of rheumatoid arthritis. *Arthritis and Rheumatism*, 9: 658–674.

Kjeldsen-Kragh, J., M. Haugen, C. F. Borchgrevink, et al. 1991. Controlled trial of fasting and one-year vegetarian diet in rheumatoid arthritis. *Lancet*, 338: 899–902.

17. Self and Nonself

Burnet, M. 1970. *Self and Not-Self*. Melbourne: Melbourne University Press.

Dausset, J. 1984. The birth of MAC. *Vox Sanguinis*, 46: 235–237.

Hamilton, D. 1982. A history of transplantation. In *Tissue Transplantation*, ed. P. J. Morris, pp. 1–13. Edinburgh: Churchill-Livingstone.

Medawar, P. 1986. *Memoir of a Thinking Radish*. Oxford: Oxford University Press.

Murphy, J. B. 1926. *The Lymphocyte in Resistance to Tissue Grafting, Malignant Disease, and Tuberculous Infection: An Experimental Study*. New York: Rockefeller Institute for Medical Research, monograph no. 21.

18. The Race for Answers

Aho, K., P. Ahvonen, A. Lassus, et al. 1974. HL-A 27 in reactive arthritis: a study of Yersinia arthritis and Reiter's disease. *Arthritis and Rheumatism*, 17:521–526.

Bluestone, R. 1985. Identification of associations with HLA-B27. In *Milestones in Rheumatologic Patient Care, 1965–1985*, ed. J. F. Fries. Syntex Laboratories.

Brewerton, D. A. 1976. Joseph J. Bunim memorial lecture: HLA-B27 and the inheritance of susceptibility to rheumatic disease. *Arthritis and Rheumatism*, 19:656–668.

Tiwari, J. L., and P. I. Terasaki. 1985. *HLA and Disease Associations*. New York: Springer-Verlag.

19. DNA, RNA, and Proteins

Bracewell, R. N. 1989. The Fourier transform. *Scientific American*, 260: 62–69.

Bragg, L. 1943. *The History of X-ray Analysis*. London: Longmans Green.

Kendrew, J. C. 1961. The three-dimensional structure of a protein molecule. *Scientific American*, 205: 96–110.

Olby, R. 1974. *The Path to the Double Helix*. London: Macmillan.

Pauling, L. 1963. The genesis of ideas. In *Proceedings of the Third World Congress of Psychiatry, 1961*. Toronto: University of Toronto Press.

Perutz, M. 1964. The haemoglobin molecule. *Scientific American*, 211: 64–76.

Richards, F. M. 1991. The protein folding problem. *Scientific American*, 264: 34–41.

20. The Beauty of Crystals

Bjorkman, P. J., M. A. Saper, B. Samraoui, et al. 1987. Structure of the human class I histocompatibility antigen, HLA-A2. *Nature*, 329: 506–512.

Madden, D. R., J. C. Gorga, J. L. Strominger, et al. 1991. The structure of HLA-B27 reveals nonamer self-peptides bound in an extended confirmation. *Nature*, 353: 321–325.

Sanderson, A. R. 1968. HLA substances from human spleens. *Nature*, 220: 192–195.

21. Cells in Action

Unanue, E. R., and P. J. Allen. 1987. The basis for the immunoregulatory role of macrophages and other accessory cells. *Science*, 236: 551–557.

Werdelin, O. 1987. Determinant protection: a hypothesis for the activity of immune response genes in the processing and presentation of antigens by macrophages. *Scandinavian Journal of Immunology*, 24: 625–636.

22. Truth Is Rarely Simple

Brewerton, D. A. 1984. A reappraisal of rheumatic diseases and immunogenetics. *Lancet*, ii: 799–802.

Voluntary Health Organizations

Some readers will know that they have one of the diseases described in this book. Whether or not they are receiving medical treatment, they will be seeking practical advice and help. In most countries of the world there are nonprofit organizations that provide services, social activities, advice, and education for people with arthritis and their families. Most of these groups work for all who have arthritis, and they campaign with government and other public bodies to improve every aspect of arthritis care. Many of the organizations fund research—especially into the causes of arthritis.

As examples, listed below are organizations in the United States, Canada, and Britain that deal with all types of arthritis. In addition, many specialized societies have been set up to benefit people with particular disorders, such as ankylosing spondylitis, back pain, juvenile arthritis, lupus, osteoporosis, psoriasis, or systemic sclerosis.

Individuals who suffer from arthritis are invited to contact organizations in their country. The various groups work together, and any of them will tell you if a different society would be more appropriate for you.

As in all nonprofit health organizations, there is always a shortage of volunteers, facilities, and funding to provide sufficient aid for either the people in need or the fight against arthritis. Support, in whatever form, is much appreciated.

ARTHRITIS FOUNDATION
1314 Spring Street, N.W., Atlanta, Georgia 30309 (national headquarters); or P.O. Box 19000, Atlanta, GA 30326; telephone 1-800-283-7800

The Arthritis Foundation funds research to find the cure for arthritis and to prevent it, and through a variety of services seeks to improve the quality of life of those affected by arthritis. The foundation is the only national, voluntary health organization in the United States that works for all people affected by the many forms of arthritis or related diseases. Volunteers in chapters nationwide help to support research, professional and community education programs, services for people with arthritis, government advocacy, and fundraising activities.

Two specialized groups exist under the Arthritis Foundation umbrella. The Arthritis Health Professions Association comprises physical and occupational therapists, nurses, social workers, physicians, and other health professionals interested in the treatment of arthritis. The American Juvenile Arthritis Organization is a council of the Arthritis Foundation composed of children, parents, teachers, and other concerned specifically with juvenile arthritis.

Arthritis Foundation nationwide services include:

Free booklets containing information about the different types of arthritis, medications, treatments, and tips for coping with daily activities.

Support for research on specific types of arthritis and research questions.

Volunteers who work with local, state, and national officials to represent the needs of people with arthritis.

Arthritis self-help courses (six-week classes totaling fifteen hours) for people with arthritis, their families, and friends, to help people learn to take an active role in their own care. The courses cover medications, joint protection, energy conservation, exercises, and ways to reduce pain and depression.

Clubs and support groups that offer discussions, guest speakers, social activities, and suggestions on how to overcome problems caused by arthritis, and that provide encouragement and support for people by sharing their problems and successes with others in the group.

Aquatics exercise programs (of six to ten weeks) in a heated pool to increase range of joint motion, reduce pain, and minimize joint stress.

Exercise programs graded for people of varying physical ability and age, and videotapes to help them continue exercising at home.

Videotapes to educate people on how to fight arthritis and to teach individuals positive ways to cope with their disease.

One-session forums for the public to have questions answered by local experts. Meetings may include workshops and demonstrations of how to take a more active role in arthritis care. A speakers' bureau arranges for local speakers to talk about arthritis issues to civic groups and other gatherings.

Lists of local doctors who specialize in treating arthritis; lists of other local resources such as special equipment.

Arthritis Today, a bimonthly magazine that brings news about arthritis research and treatments, gives tips on how to cope with arthritis, and tells stories of those living with the disease.

ARTHRITIS SOCIETY
250 Bloor Street, E Ste 401, Toronto, Ontario, M4W 3P2, Canada;
telephone (416) 967-1414; fax (416) 967-7171.

The Arthritis Society is the only nonprofit organization in Canada devoted solely to funding arthritis research, patient care, and public education. The general public is informed via pamphlets and telephone messages.

A quarterly magazine, *Arthritis News,* provides subscribers with up-to-date information about arthritis and various ways to cope with the disease.

ARTHRITIS AND RHEUMATISM COUNCIL
Copeman House, St. Mary's Court, St. Mary's Gate,
Chesterfield, Derbyshire, S41 7TD, England;
telephone (0246) 558033; fax: (0246) 558007.

More than any comparable organization, the Arthritis and Rheumatism Council concentrates on funding research into the causes and cure of arthritis.

The council also produces a wide range of publications, including more than thirty booklets for patients. Each explains a particular form of arthritis or offers practical advice on coping with the disease. There are also information sheets and videotapes on specific aspects of arthritis.

Arthritis Today, a magazine for people with arthritis, is published three times a year.

ARTHRITIS CARE
18 Stephenson Way, London NW1 2HD, England;
telephone (071) 916-1500.

Arthritis Care helps people with arthritis to help themselves, through a wide range of positive services. These include a welfare department that deals with more than two thousand letters and phone calls a month; 540 branches that provide support, information, education, social activities, and fun for sixty thousand members; and a network of 175 volunteers who visit thousands of virtually housebound individuals. Young Arthritis Care is a rapidly growing national self-help group for younger people who have arthritis.

Arthritis Care distributes practical leaflets about arthritis and its management; runs specially adapted Arthritis Care hotels and self-catering units that enable more than ten thousand people with arthritis a year to have a holiday; publishes an informative quarterly newspaper, *Arthritis News,* with a circulation of over one hundred thousand.

In addition, Arthritis Care speaks for people with arthritis, representing their concerns and their views to national government departments, local government authorities, and public bodies of all kinds.

Acknowledgments

After a professional lifetime in medicine, much of it spent in the study of diseases of joints, I find it impossible to attribute my knowledge and thoughts to specific people or specific sources of information. I am uniquely indebted to an immense number of people—especially my patients, their relatives, and many friends who have taught me the realities of living with a physical disability.

In the preparation of this book, the librarians at Westminster Hospital and at the Royal Society of Medicine were extraordinarily patient and helpful in seeking out the relevant literature, including some dust-laden elderly volumes. Toby Robertson and Reinhart Wentz gave invaluable help with translation whenever I needed it. The staff of the Department of Medical Illustration of Charing Cross and Westminster Medical School went to endless trouble to assist me with the illustrations, as did David Brady at the Wellcome Institute for the History of Medicine.

I am especially grateful to the following people for their unstinting advice and information: Kimmo Aho, Erik Allander, Rodney Bluestone, David Caughey, Leslie Courtright, Jean Dausset, Carson Dick, Paul Doury, Ronald Jubb, Marcel Kahn, Andrew Keat, Alexander Kennaway, William Kuzell, Stafford Lightman, Sam McGee-Russell, Pamela Murray, Richard Rees, Arnold Sanderson, Sydney Selwyn, Allen Steere, Joseph Stratford, Jack Strominger, Paul Terasaki, Ole Werdelin, Nick Wide, Don Wiley, and Robert Winchester. Pamela Bjorkman's detailed account of her exciting work on the three-dimensional structure of HLA molecules was an outstanding contribution.

The figures (all but two) were originally drawn by me. But I am no artist, and I am deeply indebted to Linda Forman for transforming my sketches into such high-quality artwork.

My thanks are extended also to those who kindly gave permission for use of the illustrations that appear in the text: the Wellcome Institute for the History of Medicine—pages 15, 17, 23, 26, 29, 31, 33, 78, and 96; the Medical Society of London—page 57; Ilkka Paronen—page 58; Allen Steere—page 66; Robert Winchester—page 81; the Moravské Museum—page 112; the McGill University Archives—page 155; the Mayo Foundation—page 157; Jonas Kellgren—page 188; Jean Dausset—page 204; the Department of Medical Illustration of Charing Cross and Westminster Medical School—pages 209 and 211; Peter Stastny—page 221; Pamela Bjorkman—pages 239 and 248; and Emil Unanue—page 253.

Over the past months I have become good friends with Howard Boyer and Vivian Wheeler, both of Harvard University Press. I have greatly admired their knowledge of books and their skill with the English language; and I hope that they have enjoyed learning more about medicine. It has been a privilege and a pleasure to work with the staff of Harvard University Press.

Most of all, I thank my wife, Joan, for her continuing support and invaluable advice.

Index

ABO blood groups, 198
Acquired immunity, 202–203
Acromegaly, 132
Addison, Thomas, 152–153
Adrenal glands, 152–160
Adrenal hormones, 152–160
Adrenaline (epinephrine), 153, 154, 160
Africa, 193, 272
Afzelius, Arvid, 67
Age of onset, 90, 101–102, 121, 262, 265; for different types of arthritis, 136–140; reasons for differences in, 139–140, 258
AIDS, 80–82, 224, 266, 273
Air pollution, 194, 267–268, 273
Alaska, 220
American Rheumatism Association, 213
Amiel, J. L., 206, 207
Amino acids, 227, 228, 229, 230
Anatomy: of joints, 39–42; of spinal cord, 162–163
Anemia, 92
Ankylosing spondylitis, 88–89, 91, 92, 93, 141, 180, 279; age of onset, 137–138; defined, 279; environmental triggers and, 192; first descriptions of, 98–99; geographic distribution of, 190; heredity and, 191; HLA molecule and, 208–213, 219, 220, 222; overlap and, 89, 90–91, 215–217
Anthrax, 18
Antibodies, 32, 34, 35, 38, 204–207. *See*
also Autoimmunity; Humoral immunology
Antigen-presenting cells, 38, 221, 252–256
Antigens, 32, 34, 35, 37; body's defenses against, 71–72; external vs. internal, 250–251, 254–255, 256; HLA, 205–207; number of, 38, 256; response of cells to, 250–258; transport of, 72–76
Antitoxin, 31–33
Archer, Benjamin, 130
Arthritis: attitudes toward, 2–3, 138; classification of types of, 93–94, 261–262; distribution of joints affected by, 257–258, 262; episodic, 119–120; geographic distribution of, 189–190, 219–220; hemophilic, 120; herpes and, 80; juvenile rheumatoid, 66, 137; parasite, 83–86; peripheral, 88–89, 90–91, 191, 214, 215–217; post-dysenteric, 56–59, 68–69, 89, 190, 219; sexually acquired, 56–57, 59, 68, 80, 89, 94, 191, 214, 273; systemic, 136; as term, 43–44; viral, 79–82, 140. *See also* Osteoarthritis; Psoriatic arthritis; Reactive arthritis; Rheumatoid arthritis
Arthroscopy, 50, 75, 82, 149–150
Asbestos, 194
Aschoff, Ludwig, 70–71
Aspirin, 122
Atkin, Steven, 85

DATE DUE

OCT 1 6 1994	FEB 1 9 1998	
MAR 1 4 2005		
OCT 2 3 1994	MAR 1 6 1998	
MAR 0 2 1995	JUN 0 2 1998	
	MAY 3 1 1998	
JUN 2 9 1995	APR 0 9 2000	
7/20/95	MAR 2 9 2000	
JUL 1 0 1995		
OCT 2 3 1995	NOV 2 8 2003	
MAR 1 6 1996		
FEB 2 6 1996		
OCT 1 2 1997		
	RENEWALS 362-8433	

DEMCO 38-297